P2238
2014

O A N L

OXFORD AMERICAN NEUROLOGY LIBRARY

Parkinson's Disease

Dr. Hawley and Dr. Cook are medical officers in the United States Armed Forces, and Dr. Cannard is a Federal Employee within the Department of Defense. The opinions expressed in the text are the views of the authors alone, and do not necessarily reflect the views of the United States Department of Defense or any other Federal Government Agency.

O A N L
OXFORD AMERICAN NEUROLOGY LIBRARY

Parkinson's Disease: Improving Patient Care

Edited by

Jason S. Hawley, MD
Assistant Professor of Neurology
Walter Reed National Military Medical Center
Uniformed Services University of Health Sciences
Bethesda, Maryland

Melissa J. Armstrong, MD, MSc
Assistant Professor of Neurology
University of Maryland School of Medicine
Baltimore, Maryland

William J. Weiner, MD
Former Professor and Chairman
Department of Neurology
University of Maryland School of Medicine
Baltimore, Maryland

OXFORD
UNIVERSITY PRESS

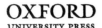

OXFORD
UNIVERSITY PRESS

Oxford University Press is a department of the University of Oxford.
It furthers the University's objective of excellence in research, scholarship,
and education by publishing worldwide.

Oxford   New York
Auckland   Cape Town   Dar es Salaam   Hong Kong   Karachi
Kuala Lumpur   Madrid   Melbourne   Mexico City   Nairobi
New Delhi   Shanghai   Taipei   Toronto

With offices in
Argentina   Austria   Brazil   Chile   Czech Republic   France   Greece
Guatemala   Hungary   Italy   Japan   Poland   Portugal   Singapore
South Korea   Switzerland   Thailand   Turkey   Ukraine   Vietnam

Oxford is a registered trademark of Oxford University Press
in the UK and certain other countries.

Published in the United States of America by
Oxford University Press
198 Madison Avenue, New York, NY 10016

Library of Congress Cataloging-in-Publication Data
Parkinson's disease (Hawley)
Parkinson's disease : improving patient care / edited by Jason S. Hawley, Melissa J. Armstrong,
William J. Weiner.
   p. ; cm. — (Oxford American neurology library)
Includes bibliographical references and index.
ISBN 978–0–19–999787–9 (alk. paper)
I. Hawley, Jason S., editor of compilation.   II. Armstrong, Melissa J., editor of
compilation.   III. Weiner, William J., editor of compilation.   IV. Title.
V. Series: Oxford American neurology library.
[DNLM: 1. Parkinson's disease.   2. Patient Care Planning. WL 359]
RC382
616.8′33—dc23
2013029039

9 8 7 6 5 4 3 2 1
Printed in the United States of America
on acid-free paper

Dedication

We would especially like to thank our families for their support and encouragement as we have worked on this textbook and during each stage of our careers.

We would like to dedicate this text to the senior editor, Dr. William J. Weiner, who passed away prior to the publication of the text. Dr. Weiner's contributions to the field of movement disorders and Parkinson's disease were innumerable. We believe the spirit of this text—dedicated to improving patient care for those suffering from Parkinson's disease—is very much in line with Dr. Weiner's remarkable career, dedicating his life as an expert clinician, educator, and advocate for improving the lives of patients with PD. As our mentor, colleague, and friend, we will miss him greatly.

Jason S. Hawley
Melissa J. Armstrong

Contents

Preface

With this volume of the Oxford American Neurology Library focusing on Parkinson's disease (PD), we sought to develop a clinically oriented, user friendly text that focuses on the basics of PD care with updates reflecting the most recent advances to the field. In developing *Parkinson's Disease: Improving Patient Care*, our goal was to provide accessible guidance to the variety of clinicians who may be involved in the management of PD patients. Our target audience includes not only general neurologists, but also others who commonly encounter patients with PD: internists, family practitioners, geriatricians, psychiatrists, rehabilitation specialists, advanced nurses, and others. As the management of PD has become increasingly complicated, a team approach is often necessary and of great benefit to patients and families. It is imperative that we all "read from the same sheet of music." In this light, we try to provide a brief guide explaining basic yet up-to-date principles along with helpful "pearls of wisdom" easily remembered and implemented.

The text can be divided into three parts. In Chapters 1 through 4, we focus on making the diagnosis of PD. We define what PD is, how to recognize it clinically, and how to distinguish it from other diagnoses. We conclude this section with Chapter 4, which aims to help clinicians understand the natural history of PD, how it progresses, and what their patients can expect. In Chapters 5 through 8, we review the management of early- to mid-stage PD. We update the reader on the rapidly expanding understanding of how non-motor symptoms are not only common and disabling in PD, but often treatable. In this section, we aim to provide concise, up-to-date strategies to identify and manage the common motor and non-motor symptoms in PD. In Chapters 9 through 12, our focus is on advanced PD, which is complex and at times an overwhelming experience for patients, families, and even clinicians. We discuss when advanced treatments like deep brain stimulation (DBS) may be helpful, and when patients benefit most from a transition to a more palliative-care approach. This section also includes a chapter on managing hospitalized PD patients—a topic often missing from comprehensive PD textbooks. Finally, we end the text by validating how ancillary specialists support the treatment of patients with PD. This includes mental health professionals and rehabilitation specialists. Our overall effort is to take the reader from beginning (diagnosis) all the way to the end (advanced PD) with a focus on the role of the clinician throughout.

The authors who contributed to the text are dedicated neurologists with vast experience in caring for patients with PD. Many have contributed significantly to the field of PD and are active in medical education both within their respective institutions as well as in national and international neurology society meetings. The contributors also have active practices where they see patients with PD daily, and they understand the day-to-day challenges for patients, families, and clinicians. Through each chapter, our aim was to extract many of the words or pearls of wisdom from our experienced contributors. We instructed our expert contributors to provide these insights in a rapidly accessible form; hence we have tried to provide tables and charts in each chapter, enabling the reader to review topics simply and easily. This is a text to be used and referenced. It can be read cover to cover or referenced rapidly in the hallway for quick guidance between patient visits.

Jason S. Hawley
Melissa J. Armstrong
May 6, 2013

Contributors

Kevin R. Cannard, MD

Associate Professor of Neurology
Walter Reed National Military
   Medical Center
Uniformed Services University
   of Health Sciences
Bethesda, Maryland

Kelvin L. Chou, MD

Thomas H. and Susan C. Brown Early
   Career Professor in Neurology
University of Michigan Medical
   School
Ann Arbor, Michigan

Barbara S. Connolly, MD

Department of Medicine Division
   of Neurology
Toronto Western Hospital
University of Toronto
Toronto, Ontario, Canada

Glen A. Cook, MD

Department of Neurology
Walter Reed National Military
   Medical Center
Bethesda, Maryland

Connie Marras, MD, PhD

Assistant Professor of Neurology
Toronto Western Hospital
University of Toronto
Toronto, Canada

Janis Miyasaki, MD, MEd, FRCPC

Associate Clinical Director
The Movement Disorders Centre
Associate Professor of Neurology
University of Toronto
Toronto Western Hospital
Toronto, Canada

Stephen G. Reich, MD

The Frederick Henry Prince
   Distinguished Professor in
   Neurology
Department of Neurology
University of Maryland School of
   Medicine
Baltimore, Maryland

Binit B. Shah, MD

Assistant Professor of Neurology
University of Virginia
Charlottesville, Virginia

Jennifer Singerman, MD, FRCPC

Department of Neurology
Sunnybrook Health Sciences Centre
Toronto East General Hospital
Toronto, Ontario, Canada

Michael J. Soileau, MD

Department of Neurology
University of Texas Health Science
   Center in Houston
Houston, Texas

x

Chapter 1

What Is Parkinson's Disease?

Jason S. Hawley

Parkinson's disease (PD) is a common neurological disorder with a significant impact on society, individuals, and families. It is a slowly progressive neurodegenerative syndrome affecting movement and gait function in the early to mid-stages of the disease, and cognitive function in the later years of the disease. Patients with PD are treated in both primary care and subspecialty care settings in all stages of the disorder. As it is often considered a "waiting room diagnosis," many individuals with PD are diagnosed (or at least suspected of diagnosis) by their primary care physician. Early medical treatment is commonly initiated in primary care, and as PD is such a common disorder among the elderly, many primary care physicians have gained experience in recognizing, diagnosing, and using several medical treatments for their patients with early PD.

Over the past two decades, neurologists and subspecialty trained *movement disorder* neurologists have rapidly expanded the menu of treatment options for PD and related complications. As the disease progresses and complications arise, patients inevitably require subspecialty care and treatment. In the later stages of PD, even the most advanced measures fail to relieve disabling symptoms, and the management becomes centered on palliative care. Throughout the entire disease course, ancillary specialists such as physical therapists, speech therapists, and mental health professionals play pivotal roles in assisting in the care of patients with PD.

Parkinson's disease holds the distinction as the only neurodegenerative disorder for which a meaningful treatment exists. The main neuropathological feature of the disease is the relentlessly progressive loss of neurons starting in the brainstem and progressing to the cerebral cortex.[1] The cardinal clinical features of PD include an asymmetrical resting tremor, slowness of movement, increased muscular tone, and instability in gait and posture.[2] While there is no current treatment that stalls this process, many of the motor symptoms can be treated with medications and procedures that activate dopamine receptors within the brain. It is also clear that in treating the motor symptoms of PD, it is possible to forestall functional disability and dramatically improve mortality.[3] Prior to the discovery of levodopa in patients with PD, most individuals with PD died within five to ten years of disease onset. Today, with symptomatic treatments, many patients with PD can expect to live close to a normal life expectancy for their age.

As treatments for PD have advanced and individuals are living longer with PD, there is greater awareness of the complications of long-term treatment and the emergence of "non-motor" symptoms. These non-motor symptoms, such as depression, urinary problems, cognitive dysfunction, and gait freezing/falling have proven to be poorly responsive to dopamine-based therapies. Moreover, non-motor symptoms contribute significantly to overall disability and quality of life for patients with PD.[4] While neurologists and primary care practitioners frequently handle many of these problems, ancillary specialists can play important roles in assisting in the management of these non-motor symptoms. As symptom management continues to be the mainstay treatment of PD, it is clear that current management of PD involves a team approach.

Patients with PD are treated by a wide variety of clinical specialties, and the main goal of this book is to provide clinicians in primary care, neurology, and ancillary specialties a practical and current guide to diagnosing and managing PD and its complications to improve patient care. The book can be divided into three sections. Chapters 1 through 4 will cover the diagnosis of PD, a discussion of disorders that can mimic PD symptoms, and a review of the natural history of the progression of PD, using a "frequently asked questions" approach. In Chapters 5 through 8, we review the treatment options for PD, focusing on the early and middle stages of the disorder. In this section of the text, we will cover both the treatment of motor symptoms as well as non-motor symptoms. We conclude this section by a review of deep brain stimulation (DBS), surgery focusing on who benefits from the procedure and when to consider referring patients to a movement disorder specialist for consideration of DBS. In the final section, Chapters 9 through 12, we cover special situations for PD care, including unique problems of managing PD in an inpatient setting, palliative care considerations in the late stages of the disorder, and the role of ancillary specialists who can offer significant supportive services for patients with PD. Through these three sections, we aim to educate and update the entire team involved in the care of the PD patient. We will attempt to be both comprehensive and accessible, and we expect that many in our audience do not have formal training in neurology. We expect this text may serve as a readily accessible book in a medical library, a clinician's office, or even the pocket of a lab coat.

Historical Background: 1817 to Today

In 1817, James Parkinson, a general practitioner in London, published his "Essay on the Shaking Palsy" in which he described six patients who displayed the clinical features of what we now recognize as PD. Parkinson was the first to recognize that the clinical syndrome was a specific disorder, which he termed "Paralysis Agitans." He described in detail the elements of tremor, postural instability, and shuffling gait.[5]

Unfortunately, James Parkinson's description went largely unnoticed until the 1860s, when Jean-Marie Charcot brought the syndrome back to forefront of research and investigation at the Salpetrière Hospital in Paris, France. From Charcot's work to today, the core clinical features of the syndrome of Parkinson's disease have largely remained unchanged.[6]

Work throughout the twentieth century expanded the understanding of underlying pathology and neurochemistry in PD. In the early 1900s, the substantia nigra, a pigmented structure in the midbrain, was found to be the pathological substrate in patients with PD. In 1952, it was recognized that PD had a defined pathology in the brainstem, which included both the presence of degeneration within the substantia nigra as well as the presence of Lewy bodies. The cause of this degeneration remained unknown. During the 1960s, the drug Levodopa (a precursor to the neurotransmitter dopamine), was found to dramatically improve the motor symptoms of PD. Moreover, with levodopa and other drugs that stimulated dopamine receptors (termed *dopamine agonists*) treating motor symptoms in PD, patients with PD had dramatically reduced morbidity and mortality.[7]

Today, we continue to refine and expand our understanding of PD (Table 1.1). The syndrome of PD is characterized by the cardinal features of a resting tremor that initially occurs on one side of the body. There is slowness of movement (bradykinesia), increased tone (cogwheel rigidity), and changes in posture and gait (a shuffling gait with instability). For most patients with PD, motor symptoms are the dominant features early on in the disorder. The diagnosis is made clinically, based on a thorough examination and history. PD is a progressive neurodegenerative disorder with likely genetic and environment factors playing a role in its cause. We now understand that PD affects much more than the motor system. Non-motor problems such as cognitive, psychiatric, sleep, and balance symptoms have led us to view PD as a much more complex disorder. The most significant advances in the last decade have further expanded our view that PD is likely to be a combination of many different disorders. Genetic analysis has revealed several genes implicated in developing PD, and different subtypes of PD have been recognized. Identifying the heterogeneity of PD is an active area of research that will probably fundamentally change the way we view and treat our patients with PD in the future.[8]

Epidemiology

Parkinson's disease is the second most common neurodegenerative disease (Alzheimer's disease is first) in North America and Europe.[9] In 2010, there were an estimated 1.1 million individuals with PD in the United States alone. Projected estimates predict that by 2030, the number of the individuals with

Table 1.1 Evolving Concepts and Controversies in Parkinson's Disease
Defining when PD begins, identifying symptoms before the advent of motor symptoms: "pre-motor symptoms"
Role of genetics in the etiology of PD
Pursuit of a consistent biomarker for the diagnosis and progression of PD beyond the clinical assessment
Discovery of a therapy that slows the progression of the neurodegeneration of PD
Improving treatment options for motor symptoms, especially gait problems poorly responsive to Levodopa
Causes, management, and treatment of non-motor symptoms in PD

Table 1.2 Causes of Death: Comparing Individuals with Parkinson's Disease and Those Without Parkinson's Disease[12]

Cause of Death	Percent in individuals with PD	Percent in individuals without PD
Cardiovascular Disorders	21%	28%
Respiratory Causes	13.6%	14.3%
Cerebrovascular Causes	7.6%	8.5%
Dementia	4.5%	6.8%
Cancer	13.6%	24.7%
Parkinson's Disease	18.2%	0.1%
Other	21.2%	17.4%

PD in the United States will rise to 1.8 million, and 2.5 million by 2050. The incidence of PD has been challenging to determine, given different ascertainment methods; however, several studies have shown the incidence is between 16–19 per 100,000 individuals. The incidence increases with age, with fewer than 10 percent of individuals developing PD before the age of 40.[10] The average age of diagnosis for PD is between 50 and 60. Mortality among individuals with PD is only slightly increased, unless complications such as dementia occur as the disease progresses. An individual with PD diagnosed in their early 60s and treated with standard therapies will have their life expectancy reduced by two years. Moreover, the cause of death in majority of patients with PD is non-PD complications, at similar rates to those of age-matched individuals without PD (Table 1.2). It is clear, and worth discussing with patients, that most individuals with PD will die from causes other than PD.[11]

Pathology

The hallmark pathological finding in PD is cell loss within the substantia nigra of the midbrain. Approximately 50 percent of neurons are lost before patients manifest motor symptoms. These neurons project into the basal ganglia and provide dopamine (hence the term *dopaminergic projections*) to these nuclei influencing control of movement. The presence of Lewy bodies, which are inclusion bodies containing the protein alpha-synuclein found in the cytoplasm of neurons, is found in PD. There are several closely related disorders that we will discuss later that also have aggregates of alpha-synuclein. Disorders like PD associated with Lewy bodies are sometimes referred to as *synucleinopathies*. Over the time course of PD, abnormal pathology spreads to involve brainstem structures and then cortical regions, which can affect cognition and behavior. There is significant controversy over when PD actually begins pathologically, and what structures are affected before the manifestation of motor symptoms. Whether or not so-called pre-motor symptoms can be identified is one of the main controversies. In the middle to later stages of PD, structures that are not influenced by dopamine projections from the substantia nigra show pathological changes, explaining why therapies that act on dopamine pathways do not

Table 1.3 Key Diagnostic Questions to Consider a Diagnosis Other Than PD	
Is Parkinson's disease the right diagnosis?	Does the patient have an aggressive parkinsonian syndrome?
	Does the patient have another cause of parkinsonism? (e.g., drug induced, alternative neurodegenerative disorder, etc.)
	For patients with tremor, is parkinsonism present, or does the patient have a different tremor disorder—Essential Tremor, drug-induced tremor?
	Consider the possibility of psychogenic parkinsonism, especially in young individuals.

affect many of the later symptoms of PD, like cognitive dysfunction, gait freezing, and falls.[12]

Introduction to the Comprehensive Management of PD

There are two fundamental questions facing a clinician when evaluating any patient with possible PD. The first is the diagnostic question of "Does this individual have PD?" Since the confirmation has traditionally relied on the clinical examination to establish the diagnosis, the clinician needs to be ever vigilant to re-explore the diagnosis when patients have unusual symptoms or progression, especially soon after diagnosis. Moreover, over the last few years, new imaging studies have gained approval in aiding the clinician in making the diagnosis, and these tools can be useful in certain difficult cases.[13] We will cover this in depth in Chapters 2 and 3. The second question, if PD is indeed the diagnosis, is "What is the best treatment approach?" Tables 1.3 and 1.4 demonstrate the key issues for both of these questions. Since all treatments for PD are based on symptom improvement, the focus should always be on improving or maintaining quality of life and delaying disability. Even at the later stages of PD, when patients respond poorly to most treatments for PD or suffer significant side effects from many medications, management decisions are based on mitigating disability and improving quality of life. Throughout this book, every treatment discussed will focus on these issues. Finally, every individual patient has different quality-of-life goals, expectations, and needs, all of which influence how and why a particular treatment will be used.

Table 1.4 Key Treatment Goals	
What Are the Goals of Treatment?	Establishing trust and communication with patients and their spouses so that they can communicate effectively how their symptoms impact their function and quality of life.
	Reducing disability and maintaining quality of life as much as possible.
	Avoiding complications that can reduce quality of life.
	Mitigating daily or even hourly fluctuations in treatment response.
	Paying attention to and treating non-motor symptoms, including psychological symptoms common in PD.

References

1. Braak H, Ghebremedhin E, Rub U, Bratzke H, Del Tredici K. Stages in the development of Parkinson's disease-related pathology. *Cell Tissue Res.* 2004;318:121–134.

2. Jankovic J. Parkinson's disease: clinical features and diagnosis. *J Neurol Neurosurg Psychiatry.* 2008;79(4):368–376.

3. Hoehn MM. The natural history of Parkinson's disease in the pre-levodopa and post-levodopa eras. *Neurol Clin.* 1992;10(2):331–339.

4. Chaudhuri KR, Shapira AH. Non-motor symptoms of Parkinson's disease: dopaminergic pathophysiology and 464. *Lancet Neurol.* 2009;8(5):464–474.

5. Factor SA, Weiner WJ. James Parkinson: the man and the essay. In: Factor SA and Weiner WJ. *Parkinson's Disease: Diagnosis and Clinical Management.* 2nd ed. New York, NY: Demos, 2008:1–13.

6. Goetz CG. Charcot and Parkinson's disease. In: Factor SA and Weiner WJ. *Parkinson's Disease: Diagnosis and Clinical Management.* 2nd ed. New York, NY: Demos, 2008:21–31.

7. Factor SA, Weiner WJ. Timeline of Parkinson's disease history since 1900. In: Factor SA and Weiner WJ. *Parkinson's Disease: Diagnosis and Clinical Management.* 2nd ed. New York, NY: Demos, 2008:33–35.

8. Halliday GM, McCann H. The progression of pathology in Parkinson's disease. *Annals of the New York Academy of Sciences.* 2010;1184:188–195.

9. Nussbaum RL, Ellis CE. Alzheimer's and Parkinson's disease. *N Engl J Med.* 2003;348:1356–1364.

10. Twelves D, Perkins KSM, Counsell C. Systemic review of incidence studies of Parkinson's disease. *Mov Disord.* 2003;18(1):19–31.

11. Posada IJ, Benito-Leon J, Louis ED, Trincado R, Villarejo A, Medrano MJ, Bermego-Pareja F. Mortality from Parkinson's disease: a population-based prospective study (NEDICES). *Mov Disord.* 2011;26:2522–2529.

12. Halliday G, Lees A, Stern M. Milestones in Parkinson's disease—clinical and pathological features. *Mov Disord.* 2011;26:1015–1021.

13. Godau J, Hussl A, Lolekha P, Stoessl AJ, and Seppi K. Neuroimaging: Current role in detecting pre-motor Parkinson's disease. *Mov Disord.* 2011;27:634–643.

Chapter 2

Diagnosing Parkinson's Disease

Binit B. Shah

The in-life diagnosis of Parkinson's disease is exclusively clinical. Definitive diagnosis is only made by post-mortem pathological analysis. Clinical acumen and familiarity with PD features are needed for precise diagnosis and prudent patient treatment, particularly if disease-modifying therapies become available; and early diagnosis is thus critical.

Immediate and certain diagnosis is not always possible at the first clinic visit. Delaying diagnosis where no diagnosis can be accurately made is reasonable. Patients may present with "soft" signs where confounding factors such as metabolic derangements, previous stroke, or other issues may be at play, or abnormalities may be in the range of anomaly rather than true pathological change. It is important to continually reappraise existing diagnoses and follow patients' signs and symptoms over time, as this may allow PD or alternative diagnoses to "declare" themselves and enable better diagnostic accuracy in the long term.

Cardinal Clinical Features of PD

The diagnosis of PD depends upon the presence of cardinal features (Table 2.1). Postural instability is a feature of PD, though it is not usual for this to be present early. Asymmetry of clinical features is common, though symmetry does not rule out PD. While cardinal features are typically present on the most affected side, crossed findings such as rigidity being greater on one side and tremor greater on the contralateral side can be seen.

Bradykinesia

The term *bradykinesia* literally means "slowness of movement." In PD, it is used as a general term that encompasses bradykinesia, akinesia, and hypokinesia. *Akinesia* is a lack of movement, and in PD it is associated with severe bradykinesia or a general paucity of spontaneous movement. *Hypokinesia* describes small movements. *Bradykinesia* in PD is a combination of slow movements that are of small size and the absence of movement in expected situations.

Examples of bradykinesia include facial masking, hypophonic speech, decreased eye-blink frequency, lack of hand-gesturing when speaking, and changes in gait such as dragging a leg, or diminished arm swing. Testing involves having patients perform repetitive, rapid tasks such as tapping the thumb and forefinger repeatedly, pronating and supinating the hand, and opening and closing

Table 2.1 Cardinal Motor Features of Parkinson's Disease

— Bradykinesia

— Rigidity

— Tremor

— Postural instability*

*Not seen in early disease but develops with disease progression

the fist. Slowing, small amplitude, and decreased amplitude over time (decrement) indicate bradykinesia. Testing each side in isolation is important, as testing sides simultaneously obscures the assessment. When testing the more affected limb one may observe mirror movements in the resting limb.

Writing is also an important test. *Micrographia* in PD manifests as a progressive decrease in size and legibility over the course of a sentence. This contrasts with micrographia in some other atypical parkinsonian diseases where writing starts small and stays small.

Rigidity

PD rigidity can be consistent (lead-pipe), or ratchet-like (cogwheel) with passive movement of the neck or limbs. Patients must relax as much as possible for an accurate assessment of rigidity. Unlike spasticity, parkinsonian rigidity is not load- or velocity-dependent and is constant throughout the entire range of passive movement. The useful Froment's maneuver involves testing tone in a limb while having the patient perform a motor task with the contralateral limb. This accentuates rigidity and can be helpful for detecting mild rigidity.

Tremor

PD tremor is present mostly with rest, but can be seen with posture-holding after a resetting phase (tremor re-emerges with posture holding). As opposed to essential tremor (ET), PD tremor is most prominent at rest rather than with action, though there can be a lesser component of action tremor. Tremor frequency in PD is also slower than in ET, with PD tremor being 4–6Hz and ET tremor usually in the range of 7–12Hz. In some patients, particularly with young-onset disease, one may see a coarse, high-amplitude tremor with more of an action component than a rest component, but this is uncommon. Distinguishing features of PD and ET are described in Table 2.2.

Postural Instability

Primary postural instability is a cardinal PD motor feature but is uncommon early in the disease. In fact, early and prominent postural instability is a reason to consider alternative diagnoses. Patients may complain of imbalance or insecurity when performing tasks or exercising compared to their pre-disease state, but this rarely culminates in early stumbles or falls. Bradykinesia can interfere with early postural adjustments, however. Examples can include tripping on a rug due to decreased leg activation, or an inability to quickly take a stabilizing step when knocked off-balance. Primary postural instability, in contrast, is the inability to maintain balance—particularly with changes in position—due to an inability to appreciate and maintain the center of mass of the body as a whole.

Table 2.2 Features That May Be Used to Distinguish Parkinson's Disease from Essential Tremor		
Clinical Feature	**Parkinson's Disease**	**Essential Tremor Features**
Tremor	— Rest, resets with posture holding — Lips, chin more typical of PD — Frequency: 4–~6Hz — Prominent when patient walks with hands at their sides	— Posture and action. If severe, can be present at rest to a lesser degree — Head tremor more typical of ET — Frequency: variable, typically 7–12Hz — Often quiesces when walking with arms at sides
Writing	— Slow with decreasing amplitude → micrographia	— Sloppy but large amplitude
Family history	— Typically negative	— Often positive
Effect of alcohol on tremor	— May improve slightly by reducing anxiety	— Can have marked response, but not always
Face	— Loss of emotion → masked	— Normal facial expression
Voice	— Lower volume or softer → hypophonia — Tremor uncommonly affects voice	— Normal volume — Can have a vibrato, tremulous quality on prolonged note-holding
Symmetry	— Usually asymmetrical	— Asymmetrical or symmetrical
Gait	— Slow, asymmetry of armswing and step length can be seen	— Normal

Presenting Symptoms

Tremor is often the presenting complaint of PD, though rigidity or bradykinesia is also often evident on examination. Tremor is often not disabling but can be bothersome, particularly in social situations. Family members or coworkers may notice tremor even before the patient is aware of it. Additionally, family members may note changes in the patients' mood or worsening of depression or anxiety. In many PD patients, premorbid personality traits can be amplified, such as mildly anxious people becoming problematically anxious. Such mood changes can occur before the first motor symptoms of disease are evident.

Generalized weakness is another common complaint. Strength in early PD patients is usually normal, though there may be delayed activation. However, patients feel that they are weak and have decreased endurance in even routine tasks. Patients may also note increased stiffness axially or in the limbs. This may accompany decreased dexterity. Patients may note more difficulty in daily tasks such as buttoning, putting on makeup or jewelry, writing, or typing. Stiffness may be accompanied by pain, particularly in a rigid joint such as a frozen shoulder. Another common complaint is effortful movement where patients have to concentrate on moving an affected limb. This is likely to be a combination of bradykinesia and rigidity and is accentuated later in the day or with fatigue.

Sleep changes can present prior to motor symptom onset or as part of the motor syndrome. Rapid eye movement (REM) behavior disorder (RBD) is the loss of sleep atonia during dreamful sleep. Patients may speak, yell out, strike out, or throw themselves out of bed. Though patients may not be aware they are doing this, bed partners are reliable reporters of these symptoms. RBD can precede development of motor symptoms of PD by years.[1] Insomnia and frequent arousals during sleep can present at any disease stage, often associated with nocturia. Rigidity can interfere with movement in sleep, and patients may find that they cannot adjust covers easily or get comfortable in bed.

Hyposmia and anosmia can also present years before motor symptoms.[2] Patients may not notice a loss of smell so much as a change in taste (dysgeusia). Accompanying weight loss is not uncommon, in part due to this symptom. Bowel and bladder function can be affected early in the disease. Constipation is a feature of bowel bradykinesia[1] and often precedes motor features. Urinary urgency is also common, though it tends to be a complaint later in the disease course. Common symptoms and complaints in early PD are summarized in Table 2.3.

Levodopa Response

Response to dopaminergic treatment, particularly levodopa, can be helpful in strengthening PD diagnostic certainty. In one series, up to 79 percent of patients with pathologically confirmed PD had a response to levodopa rated as "good" or "excellent."[3] However, patients with PD may have difficulty tolerating levodopa, and some require higher doses to have significant benefit. PD tremor can be particularly resistant to levodopa in some individuals. Thus, lack of levodopa response does not exclude PD. Additionally, response to levodopa can be seen in atypical parkinsonian syndromes, particularly in early stages. The levodopa response in atypical parkinsonisms is usually modest and transient, however, as discussed further in Chapter 3.

Table 2.3 Common Symptoms Reported by Patients and Observers in Early PD

— Tremor
— Slow walking
— Deterioration in writing
— Generalized weakness
— Mood change
— Sleep disturbance
　　+ Difficulty turning in bed or adjusting bedsheets
　　+ REM behavior disorder
　　+ Vivid dreaming
— Decreased dexterity
— Stiff, immobile limb
— Decreased smell and/or change in taste perception

Diagnostic Criteria

Pathological Diagnosis of PD

The definitive diagnosis of PD remains pathologic. There is a loss of neurons in the pars compacta of the substantia nigra, catecholinergic and serotonergic brainstem nuclei, nucleus basalis of Meynert, hypothalamus, entorhinal cortex, and the olfactory bulb.[4] Neuronal loss in the substantia nigra causes the classical motor syndrome after 60 to 70 percent of neurons in this region are lost. Remaining cells in these areas contain ubiquitin-staining inclusions called *Lewy bodies*. It remains unclear if these inclusions are causative or a consequence of PD pathological changes.

Clinical Diagnosis of PD

The most commonly used clinical diagnostic criteria for PD were published in 1992 by the United Kingdom Parkinson's Disease Society Brain Bank[5] (Table 2.4). Other diagnostic criteria have been published, including from the National Institutes of Health.[6] Unifying these criteria is the presence of a predominantly asymmetrical syndrome of rigidity, bradykinesia, and resting tremor without atypical features such as ataxia, severe autonomic dysfunction, early falls, persistent asymmetria, history of encephalitis, repeated head injury, or prominent corticospinal tract dysfunction.

Paraclinical Testing

Imaging

Single-photon emission computed tomography (SPECT) is used to detect dopamine transporter deficiency in the striatum of PD patients. In 2011 the Food and Drug Administration (FDA) approved the radiopharmaceutical Ioflupane I123 (DaTscan) in SPECT imaging to detect dopamine transporters in the brain and distinguish neurodegenerative disorders causing dopamine transporter loss, such as PD and some atypical parkinsonian disorders, from disorders that do not, such as ET and psychogenic parkinsonism.[7] This testing does not diagnose PD, but it can be helpful if there is difficulty in distinguishing PD versus ET, for example. In the future, development of radioligands to the Lewy body or a constituent of it, the protein α-synuclein, may improve early detection of the disease. Brain computed tomography (CT) and routine magnetic resonance imaging (MRI) are unremarkable in PD; there may be nonspecific atrophy and age-related changes. Transcranial ultrasound is being studied to measure the echodensity of the substantia nigra in patients with PD. The data indicate that PD patients have hyperechoic substantia nigras compared to controls,[8] but this is not yet in routine clinical use.

Other Ancillary Tests

Currently there is a number of mutations, deletions, and multiplications of genes associated with PD. Genetic testing is not used for diagnosing PD, particularly as some individuals have mutations associated with PD without any associated symptoms. Rather, genetic testing is used to identify genotype–phenotype

Table 2.4 UK Brain Bank Society: Brain Bank Clinical Diagnostic Criteria

Step 1: Diagnosis of parkinsonian syndrome

• Bradykinesia (slowness of initiation of voluntary movement with progressive reduction in speed and amplitude of repetitive actions)
• AND at least ONE of the following:
• Muscle rigidity
• 4–6 Hz resting tremor
• Postural instability not caused by primary visual, vestibular, cerebellar, or proprioceptive dysfunction

Step 2: Exclusion criteria for Parkinson's disease

• History of repeated strokes with stepwise progression of parkinsonian features
• History of repeated head injury
• History of definite encephalitis
• Oculogyric crises
• Neuroleptic treatment at onset of symptoms
• More than one affected relative
• Sustained remission
• Strictly unilateral features after three years
• Supranuclear gaze palsy
• Cerebellar signs
• Early severe autonomic involvement
• Early severe dementia with disturbances of memory, language, and praxis
• Babinski sign
• Presence of cerebral tumor or communicating hydrocephalus on CT scan
• Negative response to large doses of levodopa (if malabsorption excluded)
• 1-methyl-4-phenyl-1,2,3,6-tetrahydro pyridine (MPTP) exposure

Step 3: Supportive prospective positive criteria for Parkinson's disease (Three or more required for diagnosis of definite Parkinson's disease)

• Unilateral onset
• Rest tremor present
• Progressive disorder
• Persistent asymmetry affecting side of onset most
• Excellent response (70%–100%) to levodopa
• Severe levodopa-induced chorea
• Levodopa response for five years or more
• Clinical course of 10 years or more

Adapted with permission, from Hughes AJ, Daniel SE, Kilford L, Lees AJ. Accuracy of clinical diagnosis of idiopathic Parkinson's disease: a clinico-pathological study of 100 cases. *J Neurol Neurosurg Psychiatry* 1992;55:181–184.

correlates and for genetic counseling, particularly in patients with young-onset disease or a strong family history.

Alpha-synuclein pathology has been demonstrated in distal colonic biopsies of patients with early, untreated PD.[9] In the future, this may provide an additional route of diagnosing PD, potentially prior to motor manifestations.

Complicating Factors

As the incidence of PD increases with age, other medical and neurological complications can confound its diagnosis. Dopamine-blocking agents, such as typical and atypical antipsychotics, certain anti-emetics (e.g. metoclopramide), and certain calcium channel-blockers (e.g. flunarizine) can cause parkinsonism and must be addressed when considering a PD diagnosis. A history of stroke, orthopedic injury, neuropathy, poorly controlled diabetes, and other diseases can lead to examination findings that make it difficult to distinguish parkinsonism from PD.

Discussing the Diagnosis with the Patient

Making a diagnosis of PD or any neurodegenerative disorder can be difficult for the practitioner and the patient. It can be difficult to find a balance between being pragmatic and maintaining a sense of hope. Many patients have seen, or will see, disabled PD patients and immediately assume that they themselves will have the same disease course. It is necessary to discourage this sort of thinking, as it is not accurate or helpful. Table 2.5 lists useful discussion points, and common questions are further discussed in Chapter 4.

Summary

The diagnosis of PD is an important step in patients' care. Early diagnosis can facilitate symptomatic treatment and improve patients' quality of life. It can also provide some relief to patients and families wondering about the reason for their symptoms. Diagnosis can be difficult when symptoms are mild or if

---

Table 2.5 Useful Points to Discuss with Patients and Families When Diagnosing PD

— If uncertain about the diagnosis, tell the patient that PD is a consideration, but there is uncertainty.

— Diagnosis is essentially clinical. There are no ancillary studies that are routinely used or useful in most patients.*

— PD is a progressive neurological disease. How it progresses and the rate of progression is not possible to predict in any individual.

— It is important to identify things that are limiting and problematic now, and address them. Dwelling on possible future issues that may or may not occur and are not preventable is unproductive.

— "Seeing other patients with PD who may be markedly disabled does not apply to you, as again it is not possible to predict how the disease will affect any particular person."

— "Reading about the disease is important, but avoid getting into a 'yet' syndrome in terms of features you read about."

*See section on SPECT-Dopamine transporter in this chapter.

complicating factors exist. It is appropriate and often necessary to utilize the specialist or subspecialist consultant to help make a diagnosis.

References

1. Postuma RB, Aarsland D, Barone P, et al. Identifying prodromal Parkinson's disease: pre-motor disorders of Parkinson's disease. *Mov Disord.* 2012;27(5): 617–626.

2. Ross GW, Petrovitch H, Abbott RD, et al. Association of olfactory dysfunction with risk for future Parkinson's disease. *Ann Neurol.* 2008;63(2):167–173.

3. Hughes AJ, Ben-Schlomo Y, Daniel SE, Lees AJ. What features improve the accuracy of clinical diagnosis in Parkinson's disease: a clinicopathologic study. *Neurology* 1992;42(6):1142–1146.

4. Lang AE, Lozano AM. Parkinson's disease: first of two parts. *N Engl J Med.* 1998;339(15):1044–1053.

5. Hughes AJ, Daniels SE, Kilford L, Lees AJ. Accuracy of clinical diagnosis of idiopathic Parkinson's disease: a clinico-pathological study of 100 cases. *J Neurol Neurosurg Psychiatry.* 1992;55(3):181–184.

6. Gelb DJ, Oliver E, Gilman S. Diagnostic criteria for Parkinson's disease. *Arch Neurol.* 1999;56(1):33–39.

7. Cataufau AM, Tolosa E, DaTscan Clinically Uncertain Parkinsonian Syndromes Study Group. Impact of dopamine transporter SPECT using 123I-Ioflupane on diagnosis and management of patients with clinically uncertain Parkinsonian syndromes. *Mov Disord.* 2004;19(10):1175–1182.

8. Prestel J, Schweitzer KJ, Hofer A, Gasser T, Berg D. Predictive value of transcranial sonography in the diagnosis of Parkinson's disease. *Mov Disord.* 2006;21(10): 1763–1765.

9. Shannon KM, Keshavarzian A, Mutlu E, et al. Alpha-synuclein in colonic submucosa in early untreated Parkinson's disease. *Mov Disord.* 2012;27(6):709–715.

Chapter 3

Atypical Parkinsonian Disorders and Other Mimics of Parkinson's Disease

Melissa J. Armstrong

One challenge particularly early in the course of Parkinson's disease (PD) is deciding whether or not a patient is presenting with PD or a PD mimic: a disease that has some features closely resembling PD but with a different cause and course. While the appropriate diagnosis often becomes apparent over time, initially the help of a specialist may be required to determine whether a patient has PD or an atypical process. At initial presentation, patients may only be labelled with "parkinsonism," and seeing their responsiveness to levodopa and the subsequent course may be needed to further guide the clinical diagnosis. Differentiating PD from its mimics is critical because some similar disorders are treatable and others carry a different prognosis than PD. Additionally, academic centers are now offering clinical trials targeting the underlying pathological changes in some of the atypical parkinsonisms (e.g. davunetide for tauopathies, ClinicalTrials.gov identifier NCT01056965), offering the only hope for some of these incurable diseases.

Atypical Parkinsonisms

The term "atypical parkinsonism" refers to a specific collection of PD-like diseases including multiple system atrophy (MSA), progressive supranuclear palsy (PSP), and corticobasal degeneration (CBD). While not technically an atypical parkinsonism, dementia with Lewy bodies (DLB) is a separate disease thought to share a spectrum with PD. General red flags for atypical parkinsonisms include rapid disease progression and a poor response to levodopa.

Dementia with Lewy Bodies

DLB is grouped with PD and PD dementia (PDD) under the broader category of "Lewy body disorders,"[1] emphasizing that these diagnoses exist on a spectrum and have underlying alpha-synuclein pathology. DLB is distinguished from PD and PDD by cognitive symptoms starting prior to or within one year of the onset of motor symptoms. In PD and PDD, cognitive complaints start more than one year after motor symptoms. While this distinction is neat on paper, many patients fall in a "gray zone."[1]

In addition to early cognitive impairment, core features of DLB include parkinsonism, fluctuating cognition, and formed, detailed visual hallucinations. Suggestive DLB features include REM-sleep behavior disorder, neuroleptic hypersensitivity, and SPECT or PET imaging showing low basal ganglia dopamine transporter uptake. Clinical features that are often present but are not proven to have diagnostic specificity include severe autonomic dysfunction, repeated falls, unexplained loss of consciousness, non-visual hallucinations and/or delusions, and depression. Various combinations of these signs and symptoms form the consensus criteria for DLB.[2] A common presentation of DLB is described in Box 3.1.

While DLB is on a spectrum with PD, DLB patients may respond less well to levodopa than those with PD.[3] DLB patients may respond better to cholinesterase inhibitors than their PDD counterparts, emphasizing the importance of trying these medications for improving cognitive function. Multiple behavioral symptoms improved in DLB patients treated with rivastigmine in an RCT,[4] and recent reports suggest that memantine, an NMDA receptor antagonist, may also be beneficial.[5,6] Because of neuroleptic hypersensitivity (a much-discussed feature, but one rarely seen), neuroleptic agents should be used with caution in DLB. Treatment with quetiapine or clozapine is recommended if needed.

Box 3.1 Case #1

A 69-year-old woman presents with a two-year history of slowing of her movements and gait imbalance with occasional falls. Her family initially attributed this to arthritis and the fact that she was getting older. Around the same time, they also noticed that sometimes she didn't seem to pay attention to conversations, while at other times she was alert and able to enjoy her hobbies, such as reading and knitting. In recent months, however, she started to describe "friends" with her in the kitchen and living room when there was no one actually there. Her husband also complained that she had started to kick and hit him in her sleep. On examination, the woman had difficulty with executive tasks. She demonstrated symmetrical rigidity and bradykinesia. She walked slowly with small steps and decreased arm swing bilaterally. She was unable to recover on the pull test and the examiner had to catch her.

Comment. PD can present with symmetrical features as in this case. However, there are several clues that this woman has something other than PD. She had fluctuating alertness dating back to the beginning of her disease course. Early cognitive impairment generally points to processes other than PD. The early imbalance and falls are also a red flag. The presence of hallucinations this early in the disease course should make the examiner immediately consider DLB as a possible diagnosis. While symptoms of RBD are not specific for DLB, they are suggestive of a synuclein-based pathology such as DLB, PD, or MSA. Overall, the described clinical picture is highly suggestive of DLB.

Box 3.2 Case #2

A 57-year-old engineer presents for evaluation because he recently fainted at work and his employer required him to have a medical evaluation. He admits that he is often light-headed, particularly when he first stands up, but this is the first time he has fainted. He has no history of cardiovascular disease, and he has not been ill recently. He also complains that he has recently been having more difficulty with sexual activities with his wife. On examination, his blood pressure when lying down is 135/70. When standing, it drops to 100/60. He is mildly stiff throughout his arms and legs, and his movements seem generally slow.

Comment. This man describes multiple types of autonomic dysfunction including OH and GU dysfunction. This history, combined with the parkinsonism seen on examination, should prompt concerns of a diagnosis of MSA-P. Symptomatic treatment of his OH and GU dysfunction can begin even as he is referred for subspecialty evaluation.

Multiple System Atrophy

Like PD and DLB, MSA is a neurodegenerative parkinsonism with alpha-synuclein pathology. It incorporates presentations previously diagnosed as *striatonigral degeneration*, *sporadic olivopontocerebellar atrophy*, and *Shy-Drager syndrome*, terms no longer used. MSA is a sporadic disease divided into two presentations, one with prominent parkinsonism (MSA-P) and one with prominent cerebellar findings (MSA-C), though overlap exists.

Clinical features of MSA include progressive parkinsonism that responds poorly or transiently to levodopa, cerebellar ataxia, dysautonomia (particularly genitourinary symptoms and orthostatic hypotension [OH]), and pyramidal signs (hyperreflexia, Babinski sign). A sample presentation is described in Box 3.2. Red flags that suggest MSA-P rather than PD are listed in Table 3.1.[7]

Referring possible MSA patients to specialists is important for evaluation, prognostic counselling, and multidisciplinary care. Autonomic function tests,

Table 3.1 Red Flags for MSA

Category	Symptoms
Early instability	Postural instability with early falls
Rapid progression	[More rapid in MSA-P than MSA-C]
Abnormal postures	Pisa syndrome (involuntary flexion of the body to one side, sometimes with rotation), disproportionate antecollis (flexion of the head forward), and/or contractures of hands and feet
Bulbar dysfunction	Severe changes in voice quality, speech, or ability to swallow
Respiratory dysfunction	Diurnal or nocturnal inspiratory stridor and/or inspiratory sighs
Emotional incontinence	Inappropriate laughing and/or crying
Modified from Koellensperger et al.[7]	

cardiovascular autonomic testing, sphincter electromyography, and magnetic resonance imaging (MRI) studies read by experienced neuroradiologists can sometimes provide further evidence for MSA (Figure 3.1).

MSA patients have reduced life expectancy (less than nine years on average, shorter than most patients with PD). Treatments for genitourinary dysfunction and OH are important to prevent complications such as recurrent infections, fainting, falls, and OH-related cognitive decline.[8] Treatments to consider for OH include increasing fluid and/or salt intake, compression stockings, and pharmacological agents (midodrine and others), but these approaches should be coordinated with cardiologists or primary care physicians in patients with cardiovascular disease given risks such as supine hypertension. Involvement of sleep specialists is important for use of continuous positive airway pressure (CPAP) to treat nocturnal stridor. Botulinum toxin injections are used for dystonia. Physical, occupational, and speech therapies may be helpful. Finally, palliative care is often beneficial as the disease progresses.[8]

Progressive Supranuclear Palsy

PSP is a progressive parkinsonism with *tau*-based pathology. Patients with PSP typically have levodopa-resistant symmetrical rigidity and akinesia, commonly lacking tremor. In contrast to PD, axial findings are usually more impaired than distal/limb symptoms. PSP diagnostic criteria require prominent postural instability with falls in the first year of symptoms,[9] though a history of falls in the first year may be absent or difficult to establish reliably. Falls in the first year are extremely rare in PD, so, if present, should immediately prompt consideration of PSP. Vertical supranuclear gaze palsy is a core feature of PSP, where patients are unable to look down spontaneously, but passive extension of the neck can achieve down-gaze. Limitation in up-gaze is insufficient for the diagnosis.

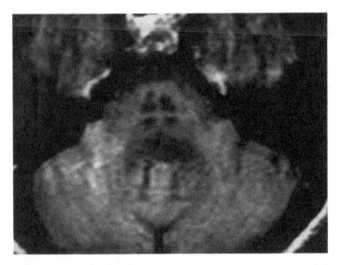

Figure 3.1 The "hot cross bun" sign in the pons is a classic MRI feature suggestive of MSA.

Specialists can often detect impairments in saccades (fast eye movements) suggestive of PSP even in the absence of frank gaze limitations.

In addition to symmetrical parkinsonism, early balance concerns and falls, and gaze impairments, common early features in PSP include having trouble swallowing, trouble speaking, cognitive impairment, and behavioral changes such as apathy. A number of clinical signs suggestive of PSP are identified (Table 3.2). A sample presentation of PSP is described in Box 3.3.

MRI can support the diagnosis of PSP if certain radiological findings such as the hummingbird sign (Figure 3.2) are present.

Patients with PSP have a median survival of eight years.[10] In addition to providing prognostic counselling, it is critical to assist PSP patients and their families in practical treatment measures, including education on fall prevention and encouragement of wheelchair use if necessary. Careful monitoring of swallowing and treatment of dysphagia is important. While pharmacological options for the parkinsonism are limited, behavioral symptoms should be treated. Speech, physical, and occupational therapy should be utilized; palliative care may be helpful in late disease stages. Clinical studies for PSP are currently recruiting, and referral to research centers is important for interested patients.

Corticobasal Degeneration

CBD is a pathological diagnosis also associated with *tau*-based pathology. The clinical presentation is now termed *corticobasal syndrome* (CBS) to emphasize that the clinical syndrome and pathological diagnosis only sometimes overlap. CBS is characterized by a levodopa-unresponsive asymmetrical parkinsonism with coexisting focal dystonia (e.g. abnormal involuntary postures in the more affected hand) and stimulus-sensitive myoclonus (rapid focal or generalized jerks in response to certain stimuli). CBS also classically has associated higher

Table 3.2 Clinical Signs Suggestive of PSP	
Applause sign	Repeated (>3) clapping after an instruction to clap three times as quickly as possible; represents perseveration and a form of frontal lobe behavior
Gunslinger sign	Wide-based gait with arms flexed and reduced arm swing
Procerus (corrugators supercilii) sign	Unusual facial expression related to procerus and corrugators contraction, reduced blinking, lid retraction, and gaze abnormalities; sometimes described as "astonished" or "worried" expression
Rocket sign	Sudden jumping to one's feet from sitting without thinking (due to frontal lobe dysfunction) only to fall backwards into the chair (due to postural instability)
Rushed micrographia	Handwriting changes early in disease onset with rapid, small handwriting from the very beginning of writing (as opposed to the progressive micrographia seen in PD)

Box 3.3 Case #3

A 60-year-old retired teacher presents for evaluation of low back pain after a recent fall. He retired two years ago because he was having more difficulty multitasking and keeping up with the demands of teaching. He has also noticed that he's having more difficulty reading. He and his wife report that he has near-falls daily and has been falling once or twice a month over recent months. His wife also complains that recently he has been crying for no apparent reason, even during happy events. When she asks him why he's sad, he denies that anything is wrong, which she finds frustrating. His signature on the clinic forms is so tiny that it's illegible. On examination, he has difficulty looking down on testing of extra-ocular movements. He has little rigidity in his limbs, but his body appears very stiff as he tries to stand. He spontaneously loses balance as he walks into the office.

Comment. The presence of early cognitive impairment, particularly in executive function given the difficulty multitasking, points to a diagnosis other than PD. The description of having trouble reading may relate more to difficulty looking down than to cognitive impairments, however. Early falls are a red flag for PSP. The involuntary and inappropriate crying likely represents pseudobulbar affect, also called emotional lability or emotional incontinence, which can be a feature of PSP and other neurological disorders. The small signature may represent rushed micrographia (Table 3.2). It is not uncommon for the rigidity in PSP to be more axial than limb.

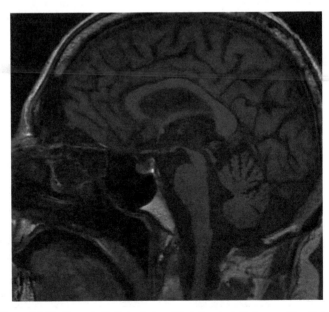

Figure 3.2 The "hummingbird" sign in the midbrain is a classic finding on mid-sagittal MRI suggestive of PSP.

Table 3.3 Higher Cortical Features Seen in CBS

Feature	Description
Apraxia	An inability to perform previously learned behaviors (not related to any physical limitation)
Alien limb phenomenon	Dissociation from one's own limb or repetitive movements of the limb outside of the patient's voluntary control
Cortical sensory loss	Sensory loss related to central dysfunction rather than the peripheral nervous system; common abnormalities include an inability to recognize a number drawn on the palm (agraphesthesia) or an inability to recognize an object by touch alone (astereognosis)
Cognitive impairment	Global deterioration in cognition with particular impairments in executive, visuospatial, and language function
Aphasia	Errors in language production and comprehension

cortical dysfunction (Table 3.3). A sample presentation of CBS is provided in Box 3.4.

Life expectancy for patients found to have CBD on pathology is 6.6 years.[11] Motor treatments are limited, but botulinum toxin injections may provide relief for disabling dystonia. Medications should be tried for behavioral complaints; agents for cognitive decline may be considered. Therapy and palliative care should be utilized when appropriate.[12] None of the atypical parkinsonisms respond to deep brain stimulation surgery.

Box 3.4 Case #4

A 64-year-old truck driver presents because he is having trouble driving due to a decreased ability to use his right hand. He has noticed over the last year that his hand has become progressively more clawed in appearance, and it is very stiff. It also occasionally jerks involuntarily. His daughter, who accompanies him to the appointment, also complains that her father has been making some mistakes when talking. For example, he may stop speaking in the middle of a sentence when he forgets the word that he wants to say, or he may say the wrong word, such as when complaining that he broke his "time" when his watch fell on the ground during a recent trip.

Comment. The patient has dystonia in the right hand with superimposed myoclonus. He also has language difficulties suggestive of aphasia. The presence of an asymmetrical movement disorder with dystonia and myoclonus and coexistent higher cortical dysfunction such as aphasia is suggestive of CBS.

Other Mimics of Parkinson's Disease

Essential Tremor

In patients presenting with tremor, essential tremor (ET) and PD are both commonly listed in the differential diagnosis, also discussed previously. Classic cases of the two diagnoses are typically simple to distinguish clinically (Table 3.4).

There are patients in whom the diagnosis is challenging, however, and a movement-disorders specialist evaluation may be required to assess for subtle signs. In cases where a clinical diagnosis is difficult to make, DaT scans may be useful. DaT scans were approved by the Food and Drug Administration (FDA) in January of 2011 for the indication of distinguishing between PD and ET, with a "positive" scan showing evidence of the brain dopaminergic dysfunction suggestive of PD. These scans are not necessary in most cases of ET and PD, but they may be useful in rare cases where the diagnosis is unclear.

Distinguishing ET from PD is important for both treatment and prognostic considerations. Medications for the treatment of tremor in ET are different from those used in PD,[13] though the effectiveness of ET medications is limited. In general, the prognosis of patients with ET is better than for those with PD, as ET may or may not progress or cause functional disability.

Wilson Disease

Wilson disease (WD) is critical to consider and diagnose in young-onset patients with parkinsonism, as it is one of the only curable movement disorders, if caught and treated early. Unfortunately, diagnosis is often delayed. WD has hepatic, psychiatric, and neurological presentations. One study reported

Table 3.4 Features Distinguishing Tremors in ET from PD	
Essential Tremor	**Parkinson's Disease**
Tremor seen most often with posture and action	Tremor seen most often at rest (though the resting tremor can re-emerge with posture holding)
Family history of tremor common	Family history uncommon
Tremor often improves with alcohol	No change in tremor with alcohol
Tremor may improve with propranolol or primidone (though tremor can be treatment-resistant)	Tremor may improve with levodopa or other dopaminergic therapy (though tremor can be treatment-resistant)
Onset can occur at any age	Onset usually in late 50s or 60s
Usually affects both sides of the body	Usually affects one side of the body at beginning
Tremor most common in hands but can also occur in the head and voice; leg and chin tremors less common	Tremor most common in hands but chin and leg tremors can occur; head and vocal tremors are rare
Symptoms other than tremor rarely present	Symptoms other than tremor present and may include decreased arm swing, decreased facial expression, rigidity, and bradykinesia

that 17.3 percent of WD patients presented with parkinsonism.[14] In WD cases with neurological presentations, 66 percent had rigidity and 58 percent had bradykinesia. Dysarthria, gait abnormalities, and dystonia were also common.[15] Screening for WD should be performed with serum ceruloplasmin and urine copper levels; serum copper levels are not helpful. Ophthalmological evaluation can demonstrate Kayser-Fleischer rings. Confirmation of WD can include genetic testing for ATP7B mutations and/or liver biopsy with copper measurements. MRI may help distinguish early-onset extrapyramidal disorders.[16]

If untreated, WD progresses to severe neurological disability and/or hepatic failure and ultimately, death. Treated WD patients have a normal life expectancy. Pharmacological options include penicillamine, trientine, zinc acetate, and tetrathiomolybdate, each of which has advantages and disadvantages and should be prescribed by a specialist.[14] Hepatic transplantation is an option in some circumstances. Chronic treatment prevents further decline and may also allow for neurological improvement in some individuals.

Drug-Induced Parkinsonism

Certain medications can cause features of parkinsonism or worsen pre-existing PD (Table 3.5). Such medication effects can occur at any age, but are more common in people who are 60 years old or older. All three cardinal features of PD—rigidity, resting tremor, and slowness (akinesia/bradykinesia)—can be present in drug-induced parkinsonism.[17] In a French study, central dopaminergic agents, primarily the typical and atypical neuroleptics, accounted for approximately half of cases of drug-induced parkinsonism. Another 8 percent were related to antidepressants, 5 percent to calcium channel blockers, 5 percent to peripheral dopaminergic antagonists (anti-emetics such as metoclopramide and domperidone), and 5 percent to H1 antihistamines. Over a quarter of drug-induced parkinsonism cases were related to miscellaneous drugs such as valproic acid, lithium, amiodarone, and others.[17] Because drug-induced parkinsonism can improve upon

Table 3.5 Medications That Can Cause Drug-Induced Parkinsonism	
Drug Class	**Examples**
Central dopamine antagonists	Sulpiride, tiapride, chlorpromazine, fluphenazine, haloperidol, risperidone, loxapine, olanzapine
Peripheral dopamine antagonists	Metoclopramide, domperidone
Calcium channel blockers	Flunarazine, verapamil, diltiazem
Selective serotonin reuptake inhibitors*	Citalopram, paroxetine, fluoxetine, fluvoxamine, escitalopram, sertraline
H1 antihistamines	Alimemazine, aceprometazine, hydroxyzine
Other drugs	Valproic acid, lithium, amiodarone, anticholinesterase

Modified from Bondon-Guitton et al.[17]

*While selective serotonin reuptake inhibitors have been associated with parkinsonism in some publications, they are still routinely used for treatment of depression in PD, typically without any description of worsened PD symptoms

agent cessation, stopping the offending drug is critical if medically possible. If patients do not improve when the agent is stopped, intervention with PD drugs may be warranted. In patients where levodopa or other dopaminergic agents may worsen symptoms, though (e.g., schizophrenia), addition of medications for parkinsonism must be done cautiously and through a multidisciplinary team.

Vascular Parkinsonism

No features reliably distinguish vascular parkinsonism from PD, but abnormal neuroimaging findings, including discrete basal ganglia lesions or diffuse periventricular and subcortical white matter lesions, are generally thought suspicious for a vascular cause of parkinsonian features. Certain clinical features may also be more common in vascular parkinsonism compared to PD, including older age, shorter time since symptom onset, lack of a response to levodopa, symmetrical gait difficulties, postural instability, falls, and dementia. Other features that may also be more common in vascular parkinsonism include pyramidal signs, pseudobulbar palsy, and incontinence.[18] Vascular parkinsonism is a clinical diagnosis made based on these clinical features and abnormal imaging; diagnostic criteria are lacking.

Other Rare Causes of Parkinsonism

Rarely, other genetic diseases such as dopa-responsive dystonia (DRD), pantothenate-kinase associated neurodegeneration, or neuroacanthocytosis can have features of parkinsonism. Other features generally distinguish these conditions from PD and rarely do they have purely parkinsonian presentations. Normal pressure hydrocephalus (NPH), with the classic clinical triad of cognitive decline, urinary incontinence, and magnetic gait, can also be mistaken for PD. The presence of lower extremity apraxia in NPH and the absence of other parkinsonian features can help separate the diagnoses.

Conclusion

It is important to recognize that the clinical features of PD can overlap with other etiologies. Making the correct diagnosis is important for treatment and prognostic considerations. When uncertainty exists, involvement of subspecialists is prudent.

References

1. Lippa CF, Duda JE, Grossman M, et al. DLB and PDD boundary issues: diagnosis, treatment, molecular pathology, and biomarkers. *Neurology.* 2007;68(11):812–819.

2. McKeith IG, Dickson DW, Lowe J, et al. Diagnosis and management of dementia with Lewy bodies; third report of the DLB consortium. *Neurology.* 2005;65(12):1863–1872.

3. Molloy S, McKeith IG, O'Brien JT, Burn DJ. The role of levodopa in the management of dementia with Lewy bodies. *J Neurol Neurosurg Psychiatry.* 2005;76(9):1200–1203.

4. McKeith I, Del Ser T, Spano P, et al. Efficacy of rivastigmine in dementia with Lewy bodies: a randomised, double-blind, placebo-controlled international study. *Lancet.* 2000;356(9247):2031–2036.

5. Aarsland D, Ballard C, Walker Z, et al. Memantine in patients with Parkinson's disease dementia or dementia with Lewy bodies: a double-blind, placebo-controlled, multicentre trial. *Lancet Neurol.* 2009;8(7):613–618.

6. Emre M, Tsolaki M, Bonuccelli U, et al. Memantine for patients with Parkinson's disease dementia or dementia with Lewy bodies: a randomised, double-blind, placebo-controlled trial. *Lancet Neurol.* 2010;9(10):969–977.

7. Köllensperger M, Geser F, Seppi K, et al. Red flags for multiple system atrophy. *Mov Disord.* 2008;23(8):1093–1099.

8. Granata R, Wenning GK. Multiple system atrophy. In: Colosimo C, Riley DE, Wenning GK, eds. *Handbook of Atypical Parkinsonism.* New York: Cambridge University Press, 2011;27–57.

9. Litvan I, Agid Y, Calne D, et al. Clinical research criteria for the diagnosis of progressive supranuclear palsy (Steele-Richardson-Olszewski syndrome): report of the NINDS-SPSP international workshop. *Neurology.* 1996;47(1):1–9.

10. Chiu WZ, Kaat LD, Seelaar H, et al. Survival in progressive supranuclear palsy and frontotemporal dementia. *J Neurol Neurosurg Psychiatry.* 2010;81(4):441–445.

11. Armstrong MJ, Litvan I, Lang AE, et al. Criteria for the diagnosis of corticobasal degeneration. *Neurology.* 2013;80(5):496–503.

12. Boeve BF, Josephs KA, Drubach DA. Current and future management of the corticobasal syndrome and corticobasal degeneration. *Handb Clin Neurol.* 2008;89:533–548.

13. Zesiewicz TA, Elble RJ, Louis ED, et al. Evidence-based guideline update: treatment of essential tremor: report of the Quality Standards subcommittee of the American Academy of Neurology. *Neurology.* 2011;77(19):1752–1755.

14. Lorincz MT. Neurologic Wilson's disease. *Ann N Y Acad Sci.* 2010;1184:173–187.

15. Machado A, Chien HF, Deguti MM, et al. Neurological manifestations in Wilson's disease: Report of 119 cases. *Mov Disord.* 2006;21(12):2192–2196.

16. Prashanth LK, Sinha S, Taly AB, Vasudev MK. Do MRI features distinguish Wilson's disease from other early onset extrapyramidal disorders? An analysis of 100 cases. *Mov Disord.* 2010;25(6):672–678.

17. Bondon-Guitton E, Perez-Lloret S, Bagheri H, Brefel C, Rascol O, Montastruc JL. Drug-induced Parkinsonism: a review of 17 years' experience in a regional pharmacovigilance center in France. *Mov Disord.* 2011;26(12):2226–2231.

18. Kalra S, Grosset DG, Benamer HT. Differentiating vascular Parkinsonism from idiopathic Parkinson's disease: a systematic review. *Mov Disord.* 2010;25(2):149–156.

Chapter 4

The Natural History of Parkinson's Disease

Jason S. Hawley and Melissa J. Armstrong

Upon being diagnosed with PD, most patients display varying degrees of confusion, disappointment, and dread. As the average age of initial diagnosis is around 60, many patients are still working or just recently retired, and remain very active. Most patients have at least heard of PD; however, now that it has become "personal," it carries an entirely different meaning. Patients "live" with PD, and like those with many chronic diseases, develop long-lasting therapeutic relationships with their physicians. Patients look to their physician for guidance about what they should expect. It is not uncommon for patients to bring entire lists of questions that revolve around their expectations of the progression (i.e., natural history) of PD.[1] Moreover, this is time well spent. A recent survey of PD patients reveals that patient's satisfaction was very high when they spent time with their doctor and received information about PD.[2] This chapter addresses those common questions that PD patients and their families ask.

What Is Parkinson's Disease?

This is often the first and most basic question that patients have. Even if they have done research before or after the diagnosis is made, hearing it from the mouth of their doctor is necessary confirmation. It is important for patients to understand that PD is a neurodegenerative disease that progresses slowly over years. We explain to our patients that while PD affects many different parts of the brain, early on, it predominantly affects areas of brain that regulate movement, and the diagnosis is made by examination findings consistent with the motor features of PD. Introducing the idea early that cells that produce the neurotransmitter "dopamine" are significantly affected is important for patients to understand their initial treatment.

Is There a Test You Can Do?

It's important to emphasize to patients that a diagnosis of PD is made clinically, on the basis of the historical information they provide and on the examination. Studies suggest that doctors, especially specialists, do a good job at accurately diagnosing PD in patients whose diagnosis is later confirmed after death.[3] There are no blood tests or brain scans to "prove" the diagnosis of PD. As discussed in Chapter 2, DaT scans are now available in the United States for certain indications, but these scans do not prove or disprove a PD diagnosis. In situations where there is uncertainty about the cause of a tremor, they simply let the doctor know whether or not there is an observed abnormality in the transport of the chemical dopamine. If positive (i.e., if there is an abnormality), this simply indicates the presence of a disease affecting dopamine, of which PD is only one. Also, the studies involving DaT scans have many limitations. Thus, DaT scans should never be used to "prove" PD, which remains a clinical diagnosis at this time. Only an autopsy can ultimately confirm the PD diagnosis.[4]

What Is Going to Happen to Me; What Should I Expect?

While it is impossible to accurately predict the future, there is accumulating data on the clinical progression of PD. There is wide heterogeneity in the rate of progression in PD, and it should be emphasized from the beginning that all patients are different. Several factors are consistently important in determining the rate of clinical progression and disability. Moreover, it is important to understand the different metrics used for measuring the "progression of PD." We will focus on two—progression of motor deficits and progression of disability.

Motor deficits (tremor, bradykinesia, rigidity) in PD progress slowly but steadily after diagnosis. Using a standardized examination of motor symptoms in PD, the Unified Parkinson's Disease Rating Scale (UPDRS), community-based studies in treated individuals with PD show that the mean progression rate of motor deficits is about 3–5 percent per year.[5,6] Treatment with dopamine agents can slow the progression of motor symptoms. In patients untreated with dopamine therapy (those in placebo arms of dopaminergic drug trials), the progression rates of motor dysfunction approached 9 percent.[7] This introduces an important concept that patients and their physicians need to understand—treatment with dopaminergic therapy can slow progression of the disease when measured by scales rating motor deficits. This was also demonstrated dramatically when comparing the mortality of patients with PD before the introduction of levodopa to the post-levodopa era (see Table 4.1). Treatment with dopaminergic therapy therefore matters significantly in improving functioning and quality of life, and affects mortality.

Measuring overall disability and quality of life is another metric of PD progression. The World Health Organization (WHO) defines *disability* as "any

Table 4.1 Mortality in PD: Comparing Pre- and Post-Levodopa Eras[17]			
	Average duration of PD	Mortality rate for age-matched population	Mean age of death
Pre-Levodopa era	9.4 years	2.9 ×	67 years
Post-Levodopa era	13 years	1.5 ×	73 years

restriction or lack of ability to perform an activity within the range considered normal for a human being due to an impairment."[8] In early PD, most patients report little to no significant disability from parkinsonian symptoms, but as the disease progresses, the effect on disability and quality of life increases. There is no absolute correlation between the progression of motor symptoms and disability and quality of life, especially early in the disease. For example, the severity of tremor is an impairment that has little effect on disability measures. While patients have "impairments" secondary to PD early on, they develop disability about three to seven years into the disease.[9] Both motor and non-motor features play significant roles in disability, with some correlating more strongly than others. As an example, the presence of depression has a robust correlation with reduced quality of life in PD, and cognitive impairment, when present, can also play a major role.[10] Table 4.2 lists factors associated with increased disability and reduced quality of life in PD.

Taking all this together, the answer to question of "what is going happen to me" is complex, but we do have insight to individual factors that play important roles in progression and prognosis. Early in the disease (the first five years), most patients have progression of motor impairments that will respond to dopaminergic therapy. These impairments do not typically cause significant disability. It is, however, important to treat motor impairments as best as possible for patients to maintain as high of a quality of life and normal functioning as long as possible. We often tell our patients "by treating your symptoms, we prolong the disease." Over time, between years three to seven, complications such as motor fluctuations and gait impairment often arise, and their presence is often the leading edge of disability. The presence of depression, which can be seen early or before diagnosis, can have a significant role in overall disability as well. However, depression is not universal in PD, and it can and should be monitored for and treated. The overall approach to answering the question is reassuring, given that treating many symptoms related to PD will be successful.

Finally, in asking the question "what is going to happen to me," many patients may really be asking "am I going to die from this disease?" While PD does marginally increase mortality, several factors play important roles in mortality in PD. The three most prominent include older age of onset of PD, the presence of dementia, and early onset of postural instability. Parkinson's disease is not a death sentence, and for many patients, it does not play a significant role

Table 4.2 Factors Associated with Increased Disability (Motor and Non-Motor)	
Motor Features	**Non-Motor Features**
Gait impairment	Cognitive dysfunction
Falls	Psychosis
Motor fluctuations	Depression
Dystonia	Urinary incontinence
Significant bradykinesia	Sleep disorders
Dyskinesia	Poor self-efficacy
Poor response to levodopa	

in their mortality. It is useful to take a holistic approach in PD, as many of the factors that play important roles in disability such as sleep, mood, and urinary dysfunction, are not related to any of the cardinal motor manifestations of PD. In answering the question, the clinician can provide some degree of reassurance but also establish the lines of communication and trust so that patients in the future can be honest with them about their limitations and current quality of life.

Besides Problems with Tremor (Movement), What Else Does Parkinson's Disease Affect?

Tremor is the most common presenting symptom leading to the diagnosis of PD. Many patients may not notice subtle bradykinesia or gait slowing until they are examined. It is useful to review with patients that PD affects the regulation of movement, with tremor, stiffness, and slowness being the common problems. We emphasize that PD presents asymmetrically (affecting one side of the body more than the other) in the majority of patients. Ultimately, PD can affect many other bodily functions, and we find it helpful discussing with patients non-motor symptoms such as effects on sleep, bowel and bladder function, mood, cognition, and energy level. For many patients, discussing the non-motor features of PD can be enlightening. Even in early PD, patients can experience these non-motor symptoms, and sometimes these symptoms can predate the development of the motor manifestations. The diagnosis for some patients may actually help them make sense of several problems they may or may not have reported to their physicians for several years. Educating patients about various motor and non-motor symptoms at the time of diagnosis facilitates their own surveillance of symptoms as well. This can lead to earlier recognition of problems that may emerge later.

Am I Going to Become Demented (i.e., Is This Like Alzheimer's Disease?)

Depending on how much your patient has read about PD, questions about cognition may or may not arise at early visits. Many patients are not even aware of the cognitive decline associated with PD until it occurs and/or the clinician provides education on this topic. Regardless, clinicians taking care of PD patients must be prepared to discuss the occurrence of cognitive impairment in PD, as the point prevalence of dementia in PD is about 30 percent, and the cumulative prevalence of dementia is 75 percent for PD patients surviving over 10 years.[11] Additionally, 17 to 30 percent of PD patients without dementia still demonstrate at least mild cognitive impairment (MCI), with some estimates of MCI reaching higher than 50 percent. Additionally, several studies have estimated that approximately 20 percent of PD patients have MCI at the time of their PD diagnosis.[12]

While some degree of cognitive impairment is almost inevitable in PD, it is a very different form of impairment than that seen in Alzheimer's disease (AD), and this should be emphasized to patients and their families. While memory can be affected, this is usually much less severe than in AD. Executive and visuospatial problems are the most common impairments seen in PD. Early on, executive impairments may present as subtle problems, such as having increased difficulty with multitasking. Attention can also be affected and can fluctuate over the course of the day. Eventually, PD patients may experience a severe dementia affecting most cognitive domains and requiring 24-hour support. While a few of the medicines developed for AD have been studied in PD, benefits are modest at best, and these medications do not convincingly slow the progression of the cognitive impairment.[13]

Why Did I Develop PD?

Most patients do not have a readily identifiable cause for PD. There are several genetic forms of PD, and genetic testing may be useful if there is a strong family history of PD and/or an early onset of PD (before age 40). Only one gene to date, the Leucine-Rich Repeat Kinase 2 (LRRK2) gene, has been seen in sporadic late-onset PD, accounting for just 1 to 2 percent of all cases.[14] In certain populations, like in the Ashenazi Jewish population, the rates of genetic PD may higher. Environmental exposures to metals, pesticides, and chemicals have been studied as potential casual agents, with mixed results. The etiology of PD will probably continue to be understood as multifactorial with predominant genetic factors and the interplay of environmental influences.[15]

Conclusion

The questions highlighted in this chapter are common questions that patients have after the initial diagnosis of PD, and most relate to the natural history of progression in PD. These questions often arise in the second or third visit after the initial diagnosis, as the realization and implications of PD can sometimes take time to sink in. As one of my patients once reported to me, "It took me a year to realize that my life was not over." One useful approach is scheduling a follow-up shortly after the diagnosis is made, in order to monitor how patients are coping with the diagnosis, and answer these questions. Part of the role of the clinician is helping patients through this difficult time after diagnosis. This is time well spent. As a Global Parkinson's Disease Survey in 2002 showed, "satisfaction with explanation at time of diagnosis" was actually correlated with quality of life measures for patients with PD.[16]

References

1. Findley LJ, Baker MG. Treating neurodegenerative diseases: what patients want is not what doctors focus on. *BMJ*. 2002;324:1466–1467

2. Dorsey ER, Voss TS, Shprecher DR, et al. A U.S. survey of patients with Parkinson's disease: satisfaction with medical care and support groups. *Mov Disorder*. 2010;25:2128–2135

3. Hughes AJ, Daniel SE, Ben-Shlomo Y, Lees AJ. The accuracy of diagnosis of Parkinsonian syndromes in a specialist movement disorder service. *Brain*. 2002;125:861–870.

4. de la Fuente-Fernandez R. Role of DaTSCAN and clinical diagnosis of Parkinson's disease. *Neurology.* 2012;78:696–701.

5. Schrag A, Dodel R, Spottke A, et al. Rate of clinical progression in Parkinson's disease. A prospective study. *Mov Disord.* 2007;22:938–945.

6. Evan JR, Mason SL, Williams-Gray CH, et al. The natural history of treated Parkinson's disease in an incident, community based cohort. *J Neurol Neurosurg Psychiatry.* 2011;82:1112–1118

7. Jankovic J. Variable expression of Parkinson's disease: a base-line analysis of the DATATOP cohort. The Parkinson's Study Group. *Neurology.* 1990;40:1529–1534.

8. World Health Organization. *International Classification of Impairments, Disabilities, and Handicaps.* Geneva: World Health Organization; 1980.

9. Shulman LM, Gruber-Baldini AL, Anderson KE et al. The evolution of disability in Parkinson's disease. *Mov Disord.* 2008;23:790–796.

10. Schrag A, Jahanshahi M, Quinn N. What contributes to quality of life in patients with Parkinson's disease? *J Neurol Neurosurg Psychiatry.* 2000;69:308–312.

11. Aarsland D, Kurz MW. The epidemiology of dementia associated with Parkinson's disease. *J Neurol Sci.* 2010;289:18–22.

12. Aarsland D, Bronnick K, Fladby T. Mild cognitive impairment in Parkinson's disease. *Curr Neurol Neurosci Rep.* 2011;4:371–378.

13. Kehagia AA, Barker RA, Robbins TW. Neuropsychological and clinical heterogeneity of cognitive impairment and dementia in patients with Parkinson's disease. *Lancet Neurol.* 2010;9:1200–1213.

14. Gilks WP, Abou-Sleiman PM, Gandhi S, et al. A common LRRK2 mutation in idiopathic Parkinson's disease. *Lancet.* 2005;365:415–416.

15. Shulman JM, De Jager PL, Feany MB. Parkinson's disease: genetics and pathogenesis. *Ann Review Path: Mech Dis.* 2011;6:193–222.

16. Global Parkinson's disease Survey Steering Committee. Factors impacting on quality of life in Parkinson's disease: results from an international survey. *Mov Disord.* 2002;17(1):60–67.

17. Pourfar M, Feigin A, Eidelberg D. Natural History. In: SA Factor and WJ Weiner, eds., *Parkinson's Disease: Diagnosis and Clinical Management.* New York: Demos; 2008:127–133.

Chapter 5

Medical and Non-Medical Management of Early Parkinson's Disease

Glen A. Cook and Jason S. Hawley

There are many pharmacological options available for treating early Parkinson's disease. These treatments improve most of the motor symptoms of PD for many years, allowing patients to maintain good function. These medications improve tremor, bradykinesia, rigidity, and gait impairment that result from the loss of dopaminergic cells in the substantia nigra. They act by replacing or enhancing the action of dopamine within the basal ganglia. This chapter focuses on the pharmacological agents used to treat early PD and the most critical questions of when to initiate therapy, what drugs to use, and how to individualize therapy. We will also address two important controversies regarding early treatment. The first controversy is the question of toxicity from levodopa, the most important and efficacious drug in treating PD. The second controversy is whether or not any of these drugs is "disease modifying" or "neuro-protective." Finally, our focus is on the early "motor" symptoms of PD. We recognize that the non-motor complications of PD such as depression, mild cognitive impairment, and sleep disorders can be seen early in the disease course, and this will be addressed in Chapter 7.

When to Start Pharmacological Treatment?

The decision to initiate treatment for early PD is an individual one. Patient preference, symptom severity, occupational, and recreational limitations all factor into treatment decisions. It is possible in very early PD that patients may not be limited by its symptoms, and pharmacological treatment may be deferred for months. As an example, patients with a mild, intermittent, non-limited, unilateral rest tremor and very mild bradykinesia may not require treatment at all. Most patients, however, will find some of the PD motor symptoms limiting to their everyday activities, and treatment is necessary to maintain a desired level of function. The decision to initiate treatment becomes clearer when the motor symptoms of PD limit the patient's routine physical activity, such as impairment of gait function. It is important to recognize that some patients minimize impairments from early PD, or they may not realize how the motor deficits are limiting them. Finally, patients should understand the goals of treating motor symptoms. Dopaminergic therapies typically improve bradykinesia, rigidity, and gait slowing. Patients with PD who take these therapies may notice increased energy level throughout the day, improved manual dexterity, and reduction in tremor. Decisions to increase or change dopaminergic medications often depend on the efficacy of therapy in improving these symptoms as noticed by the individual, and reported to the physician.

Pharmacological Agents for Early PD

Pharmacological therapy for early PD may be considered in two categories: "minor" and "primary" medications.[1] The minor medications include the MAO-B inhibitors and amantadine. Their efficacy is limited compared to that of the primary agents in improving motor symptoms. Selegiline (Eldepryl, Zelapar) and rasagiline (Azilect) are monoamine oxidase-B (MAO-B) inhibitors commonly prescribed in early PD. Overall, the likely effect of MAO-B inhibitors is to modestly increase dopamine concentrations within the striatum by promoting dopamine release and inhibiting reuptake.

Selegiline is given as 5 mg in the morning and can be increase to a second daily dose at noon. Rasagiline was recently approved for symptomatic treatment in PD by the U.S. Food and Drug Administration and is prescribed at 0.5 mg to 1.0 mg, given in the morning. While dietary modifications are not typically necessary with the selective MAO-B inhibitors, combining these with other serotonergic medications may precipitate the serotonin syndrome.

The mechanism of action for amantadine (Symmetrel) in PD is unclear; however, there is a mild clinical effect on motor symptoms. The drug is started either daily or twice a day at 100 mg per dose, though the total dose may be increased up to 400 mg total daily. The most common side effects are mottled skin (livedo reticularis) and pedal edema. While amantadine has been available for the treatment of PD for many years, its mechanism of action as an inhibitor of glutamate NMDA receptors has been clarified more recently.[2]

The "primary" medications for PD are the dopamine agonists and carbidopa/levodopa. These medications provide more robust relief of symptoms than the above "minor" agents. They are well tolerated and appropriate as initial pharmacological therapy for PD, acting by directly increasing dopamine levels pre-synaptically (levodopa) or stimulating dopamine receptors post-synaptically (dopamine agonists). Most patients with PD will require these medications to treat symptoms upon diagnosis or within one year after diagnosis.

The newer dopamine agonists pramipexole (Mirapex) and ropinirole (Requip) are commonly used. The most common side effects of the dopamine agonists are somnolence, sudden sleep episodes, and hypotension. Patients should also be screened for and counseled about impulse-control behaviors. Additionally, dopamine agonists should not be stopped abruptly.

Levodopa is the most efficacious medication in treating motor symptoms of PD. Levodopa is converted within the brain to dopamine by DOPA decarboxylase. Levodopa is combined with carbidopa to prevent its conversion to dopamine outside of the central nervous system, attenuating the side effects of nausea and hypotension and also reducing the total amount of levodopa

needed to produce symptom relief. The standard formulation of carbidopa/
levodopa (Sinemet) is in tablets of 25/100 strength. The "25" represents the milligram dose of carbidopa, and the "100" represents the milligram dose of levodopa. Other formulations of Sinemet with elevated levodopa concentrations
are available (carbidopa/levodopa 25/250, for example). For initial treatment,
the standard carbidopa/levodopa can be initiated with the 25/100 tablet taken
three times a day. It is preferable when starting to instruct the patient to take
carbidopa/levodopa about 30 minutes before a meal to maximize its bioavailablity and effect. Patients with PD generally tolerate carbidopa/levodopa well.
Nausea can occasionally be a problem, and we recommend taking the medication with meals as an initial solution. The addition of adding pure carbidopa
(Lodsyn) 25 mg with each dose can also be effective. A controlled-release (CR)
formulation (Sinemet CR) is also available. The standard immediate release (IR)
formulation is less expensive,[3] has better bioavailablility,[4] and has more predictable interactions with meals.[5] It is important to recognize that, due to the lower
bioavailablity of CR, the levodopa dose in CR is approximately 70 percent of
the IR formulation. For example, if a patient converts from Sinemet 25/100 IR
to Sinemet CR 25/100, there will be effectively a 30 percent lower dose of levodopa in the CR. Clinical trials comparing the standard to the CR formulation
found no benefit to the latter in patients with early PD.[6,7] Carbidopa/levodopa
is also available in a co-formulation with the catechol-O-methyl transferase
(COMT) inhibitor entacapone (Stalevo). The addition of entacapone increases
the half-life of the levodopa by about an hour.[8] Similar to the CR formulation of
Sinemet, this formulation is more expensive[4] and probably has no extra beneficial role compared to standard-formulation levodopa in the treatment of early
PD, though no clinical trials have compared the two.[1] The best use of Stalevo is
treating mild wearing-off effect between doses. This is typically not a problem
for most patients with early PD. While there are several options for using levodopa, the authors recommend starting with the IR carbidopa/levodopa as the
first option. Table 5.1 summarizes the initial medication profiles discussed.

What Is the Appropriate Starting Medication in Early PD?

This is one of the most frequently asked questions among primary care physicians and neurologists in discussing the treatment of PD. The minor agents
have a role, but it is limited to treating patients with mild symptoms. Levodopa
is the most effective therapy for treating the motor symptoms of PD, and it is
generally very well tolerated. Given this background, the obvious question is
why not start levodopa in all patients with PD? The main concern with early
initiation of levodopa is the development of levodopa-induced motor fluctuations and dyskinesia. In patients with young-onset PD (before age 40), the risk
of dyskinesias and motor fluctuations while using levodopa increases with the
duration of disease, approaching 100 percent incidence after five years in these
patients.[9] However, disability caused by these dyskinesias is usually very mild.
Multiple clinical trials have shown that dyskinesias were reduced in patients
initiated on dopamine agonists instead of levodopa.[10] Once levodopa therapy

Table 5.1 Pharmacological Treatments for Early PD

Agent	Class	Typical starting dose	Common side-effects
Selegiline	MAO-B inhibitor	5 mg in the morning and again at noon	Constipation, diarrhea, drowsiness, dry mouth, mild headache, lightheadedness, vivid dreams, hallucinations, compulsive behaviors, abnormal dreams
Rasagiline	MAO-B inhibitor	0.5 to 1.0 mg in the morning	
Amantadine	Glutamatergic NMDA-receptor inhibition	100 mg once or twice daily	Lower extremity swelling, mottling of the skin, lightheadedness
Pramipexole	DA agonist	1 mg three times per day	Nausea, somnolence, dry mouth, sleep attacks, hypotension, edema, compulsive behaviors
Ropinirole	DA agonist	3 mg three times per day	
Carbidopa/ levodopa	DA precursor (plus DOPA decarboxylase inhibitor)	25/100 mg three times per day	Lightheadedness, nausea, constipation, vivid dreams

MAO-B = monoamine oxidase-B; DA = dopamine

is initiated, dyskinesias will manifest on the same time course, as if there were no delay in starting levodopa. Thus, it is not the initiation of levodopa therapy that provokes the dyskinesia and motor fluctuations, but rather the progression of the disease with the symptoms being brought out with the levodopa dosing.[11] The initial dosing with the dopamine agonist allows the younger patient, who is expected to eventually develop dyskinesia, a greater period of time on a medication that is sufficient to treat the motor symptoms without provoking dyskinesia. Thus, in such younger patients, initial therapy with DA agonists is preferred to maximize the time without motor fluctuations or dyskinesia. In contrast, for older patients we recommend levodopa over the DA agonists due to better tolerability of levodopa and lower risk of dyskinesia in this population. Table 5.2 outlines general guidelines for initial therapy for PD.

Current Controversies in Treating Early PD: Levodopa Toxicity and Neuro-protection

Is Levodopa Toxic?

Because DA-provoked oxidative stress has been hypothesized as a cause of dopamine cell loss in PD, some have questioned whether levodopa could play a toxic role within the dopaminergic system when it is used to treat PD. This issues has been largely settled with multiple lines of evidence showing that such a "toxic" effect does not exist.[1,12] The introduction of levodopa therapy in the 1970s was followed by marked reductions in the mortality of PD.[13] The neuropathological features of PD did not change after the introduction of levodopa.[14] The use of levodopa in treating conditions besides PD has not provoked

Table 5.2 General Outline for Drug Selection in Early PD

Drug Class	Mechanism of action on DA	Expectations	Patient selection
Minor drugs (MAO-B inhibitors, amantadine)	Mild increase in dopaminergic activity	Mild improvement in non-limiting motor impairments	Early PD, minimal disability or impairment from motor deficits
DA agonists (Mirapex, Ropinirole)	Directly activates dopamine receptors	Notable improvement in motor symptoms	Patients < 60 with mild to moderate limiting symptoms
Carbidopa/ Levodopa	Directly converted to DA, increases pre- and post-synaptic DA, serves to directly replace DA within the brain	Most efficacious in improving motor symptoms	—Patients > 65 —Patients unable to tolerate DA agonists —Patients with sub-optimal treatment response from DA agonists —Patients with gait/ balance impairment, or significant motor disability

parkinsonism or findings of substantia nigra toxicity.[15] Finally, mice administered large doses of levodopa over prolonged periods (up to 18 months) do not develop substantia nigra pathology.[16] Occasionally, patients may bring up this concern, and as levodopa is invariably a treatment for all patients with PD at sometime in their disease, we recommend being clear that there is no current evidence for a "toxic" effect of levodopa.

Is There "Neuro-Protective" Therapy for PD?

A drug therapy that would slow the progression of neuronal degeneration in PD, providing cellular "neuro-protection," has been the goal of a major effort of clinical research. Unfortunately, to date, no interventions have shown to slow PD progression. To date, the concept of neuro-protection and disease modification remains challenging to patients, clinicians, and investigators. In the medication management of early PD, the authors do not currently recommend initiating a medication or supplement with the expressed benefit of neuro-protection.

Summary

A variety of pharmacological agents exists for the symptomatic treatment of early Parkinson's disease, including MAO-B inhibitors, dopamine agonists, and levodopa (combined with carbidopa). The focus of early treatment is maintaining improved motor function, and tailoring therapy to maintain the highest level of functioning in activities of daily living or employment. We provide general guidelines as a starting point for the physician starting early therapy for PD, based on patient age, motor deficits, and co-morbid non-motor symptoms.

Many patients will have questions about their early treatment, and we discuss two of the most common questions. The first, regarding the possible toxicity of levodopa, has largely been answered, and there is no current clear evidence showing a detrimental or toxic effect from the regular use of levodopa. Levodopa continues to be the most important and efficacious medication for PD. The second controversy, whether certain therapies provide a degree of cellular "neuro-protection," is harder to address. While this remains controversial, to date, it does not appear that any current medical treatment can slow the progression of neurodegeneration of PD, and treatment of motor symptoms in early PD remains focused on symptom and quality of life improvement.

References

1. Ahlskog JE. Symptomatic treatment approaches for early Parkinson's disease. In: Weiner WJ, Factor SA, eds. *Parkinson's Disease—Diagnosis and Clinical Management.* 2nd ed. New York: Demos Medical Publishing; 2007:633–641.

2. Greenamyre JT, O'Brien CF. N-methyl-D-aspartate antagonists in the treatment of Parkinson's disease. *Arch Neurol.* 1991;48(9):977–981.

3. Ahlskog JE. *The Parkinson's Disease Treatment Book: Partnering with Your Doctor to Get the Most from Your Medications.* New York: Oxford University Press; 2005.

4. Yeh KC, August TF, Bush DF, et al. Pharmacokinetics and bioavailability of Sinemet CR: a summary of human studies. *Neurology.* 1989;39(11 Suppl 2):25–38.

5. Nutt JG, Woodward WR, Hammerstad JP, Carter JH, Anderson JL. The "on-off" phenomenon in Parkinson's disease: relation to levodopa absorption and transport. *N Engl J Med.* 1984;310(8):483–488.

6. Koller WC, Hutton JT, Tolosa E, Capilldeo R. Immediate-release and controlled-release carbidopa/levodopa in PD. *Neurology.* 1999;53(5):1012–1019.

7. DuPont E, Andersen A, Boas J, et al. Sustained-release Madopar HBS compared with standard Madopar in the long-term treatment of de novo Parkinsonian patients. *Acta Neurol Scand.* 1996;93(1):14–20.

8. Holm KJ, Spencer CM. Entacapone: a review of its use in Parkinson's disease. *Drugs.* 1999;58(1):159–177.

9. Van Gerpen JA, Kumar N, Bower JH, et al. Levodopa dyskinesia risk among Parkinson's disease patients in Olmsted County, Minnesota, 1976–1990. *Arch Neurol.* 2006;63(2):205–209.

10. Rascol O, Brooks D, Korczyn AD, et al. A five-year study of the incidence of dyskinesia in patients with early Parkinson's disease who were treated with ropinirole or levodopa. *N Engl J Med.* 2000;342:1484–1491.

11. Cedarbaum JM, Gandy SE, McDowell FH. "Early" initiation of levodopa treatment does not promote the development of motor response fluctuations, dyskinesias or dementia in Parkinson's disease. *Neurology.* 1991;41(5):621–629.

12. Agid Y, Ahlskog E, Albanese A, et al. Levodopa in the treatment of Parkinson's disease: a consensus meeting. *Mov Disord.* 1999;14(6):911–913.

13. Sweet RD, McDowell FH. Five years' treatment of Parkinson's disease with levodopa: therapeutic results and survival of 100 patients. *Ann Intern Med.* 1975;83(4):456–463.

14. Yahr MD, Wolf A, Antunes J-L, et al. Autopsy findings in Parkinsonism following treatment with levodopa. *Neurology.* 1972;22(Suppl):56–71.

15. Parkkinen L, O'Sullivan SS, Kuoppamaki M, et al. Does levodopa accelerate the pathological process in Parkinson's disease brain? *Neurology.* 2011;77(15):1420–1426.

16. Sahakian BJ, Carlson KR, De Girolami U, Bhawan J. Functional and structural consequences of long-term dietary L-dopa treatment in mice. *Commun Psychopharmacol.* 1980;4(2):169–176.

Chapter 6

Motor Fluctuations and Dyskinesia: What Are They, and How Do You Treat Them?

Kevin R. Cannard

Invariably, as Parkinson's disease advances, patients develop motor fluctuations and dyskinesias. Together, these are sometimes called "motor complications." This is primarily a consequence of chronic levodopa treatment, which all PD patients eventually require. Initially, motor complications present only a minor inconvenience to the patient, but for many, motor fluctuations and dyskinesia evolve to become major contributors to their disability. As the disease progresses, the effective management of these problems can become the major focus of the treatment of motor symptoms. Fortunately, there is usually a predictable and natural progression of these complications that can be anticipated and addressed with relatively simple treatment strategies.

What Are Motor Fluctuations and Dyskinesias?

"Motor fluctuations" are unwanted clinical responses to medication dosing, usually resulting in a failure of medication to allow effective movement. These are manifested as a worsening of the classic parkinsonian features of tremor, reduced speed and amplitude of movement, stiffness and rigidity (often perceived by the patient as weakness), and gait problems. The most common motor fluctuations are a shortening of response time or unpredictable medication response times. The different types of fluctuations typically appear sequentially in a somewhat predictable pattern. Dyskinesias are the intrusions of unwanted, involuntary movements and exist in two primary forms: choreiform dyskinesias and dystonic posturing. Even though dyskinesias often present first, initially they are often so subtle as to go unrecognized by the patient and may produce little or no impairment. It is usually motor fluctuations that first interfere with functioning. It is typical that both of these motor complications eventually need to be managed. In this chapter will review how to recognize each of these motor complications, review the medications used in their management, and then explore specific strategies that can be employed to effectively control them.

Dyskinesias

Choreiform Dyskinesias

Often referred to simply as "dyskinesia," choreiform dyskinesias are the most common form of dyskinesias and consist of random, curvilinear movements that may affect the limbs, head and neck, or trunk. Patients appear fidgety and, when the condition is severe, may appear to be in constant chaotic motion. Dyskinesias tend to momentarily intensify when the patient attempts to speak or move. Anxiety may also heighten the effect. This state is usually a *peak-dose effect* of "too much" medication producing a surge of stimulation through the motor pathways, preventing the normal inhibition of unintended movements. Less commonly, "biphasic dyskinesias" may occur where patients have the extra movements as their medications are kicking in or wearing off, as opposed to at peak dose. While these movements often cause great concern among family, friends, and caretakers, most patients are surprisingly undisturbed by dyskinesias. It is only in the more advanced states when dyskinesias begin to intrude substantially into purposeful movement or affect their gait that treatment is actually necessary. Some degree of dyskinesia may be an unavoidable accompaniment of "on" states (see below), and a physician must resist the temptation to suppress them at the expense overall movement. The vast majority of patients would rather be in an "on" state with dyskinesias than entombed within a rigid, akinetic (motionless) body in an "off" state without dyskinesias. My advice is to treat the patient, not the anxiety of those around them!

Dystonic Posturing

By contrast, dystonia is a state in which a limb or body part assumes a particular posture due to the involuntary co-contraction of antagonistic muscles. Dystonia is typically a *low-dose effect*. Off-period dystonia is most commonly seen, often presenting as a morning phenomenon with foot inversion and toe flexion upon awakening when patients are at their lowest daily medication levels. It can disrupt morning mobility and may be painful. This is may be the initial dyskinesia noticed by patients, affecting the foot on the more parkinsonian side.

Motor Fluctuations

Motor fluctuations consist of the variable ability to execute voluntary movement throughout the day. In their broadest extremes they consist of *"on" periods* where a patient has full or nearly normal control of movement and *"off" periods* during which the patient experiences a return of bradykinesia (slowness), akinesia (a lack of movement), rigidity, tremor, and/or gait and postural disturbances. The Parkinsonian off states may dramatically impair a patient and even produce pain. The main motor fluctuations are noted in Table 6.1.

Why Do Motor Fluctuations and Dyskinesia Occur?

The causes of motor fluctuations are complex and beyond the scope of this chapter, but are primarily a consequence of levodopa treatment. This may be related to the very short half-life of levodopa (~90 minutes) which induces

Table 6.1 Clinical Presentations and Subtypes of Motor Complications

MOTOR COMPLICATIONS

End-of-dose "wearing off"	The anti-parkinsonian motor effects are lost prior to the next dose, causing the return of the parkinsonian state, producing **on periods** of good PD motor control alternating with **off periods** of exaggerated parkinsonian motor features.
Peak dose dyskinesias	On periods are associated with dyskinesias as levodopa/dopamine levels reach their highest serum and brain concentrations.
Morning (or nocturnal) "off" periods	Morning or nocturnal dystonic posturing or when medication levels reach their lowest point.
"On-off" phenomenon	Less predictable alternations between on and off periods that do not seem to correlate well with the patient's dosing schedule.
Diphasic dyskinesias	Dyskinesias that appear at the beginning and end of a dose cycle as levels rise and fall.
Dose failures or "delayed on"	A total lack of or greatly delayed motor response to a particular dose of medication in a patient that is otherwise responsive to the medication.
"Super-off"	This is an incapacitating state of near complete inability to move that may last from minutes to up to an hour or more.
Freezing	This is a form of "motor block" where an intended movement fails. It usually refers to freezing of gait, which prevents the patient from walking or moving for seconds to minutes.

some type of neuronal reorganization.[1] Dopamine agonists are much less likely to cause motor complications,[2] and this may be a consequence of their longer half-lives (6–12 hours). By four to six years of treatment with levodopa, the risk of developing motor fluctuations or dyskinesia is approximately 40 percent for each.[3] If one looks closely, a substantial percent of patients develops at least subtle dyskinesias within the first one to two years.[4,5] A good rule of thumb is a 10 percent per year risk of motor complications while on levodopa, and they are more common in younger patients.[6]

Treatment Strategies

Motor Fluctuations

The overall goal of treating motor fluctuations is to provide enough dopamine replacement therapy (DRT) to allow effective movement while avoiding excessive levels of medication that produce incapacitating dyskinesias (Table 6.2). This range of optimal dosing is called the *therapeutic window*. When medication dosing levels fall below this optimal range, the patient experiences excessive slowness, rigidity, severe tremor, dystonic postures, gait impairment, or even a complete failure of movement. Levels above this range result in intrusive dyskinesias, which can be incapacitating when severe. Unfortunately, as the disease progresses, there are fewer functional dopamine-producing cells in the substantia nigra, and this window progressively narrows.

In general, physicians should focus solely on functional improvements, ignoring the cosmetic effects of choreiform dyskinesias unless they significantly

Table 6.2 Treatment Approachs to managing Motor Fluctuations

TREATMENT OF MOTOR FLUCTUATIONS

End of dose "wearing off"	**Goal:** Extend the effects DRT to compensate for the loss of the storage effect that produces shorter periods of levodopa motor benefit.
	Actions to take: • **Shorten the levodopa dosing interval:** First step: decrease the dosing interval to 4 hours and eventually as short as 2. • **Add a low dose of a dopamine agonist** (has a longer $t_{1/2}$): This may not be tolerated in elderly/advanced PD patients. • **Add a COMT-I:** This may allow decreasing levodopa by 25%–30% while sustaining the motor effect.[7,8] • **Add an MAO-B inhibitor:** Effective and well tolerated.[9,10,11]
Morning (or nocturnal) "off" periods	**Goal:** Provide enough DRT to make morning hours or arising at night to toilet safe and comfortable.
	Actions to take: • **Bedside morning dosing.** • **Add a bedtime dose of controlled-release levodopa.** • **Add a rotigatine patch to the regimen:** Apply at bedtime. Caution: may cause orthostatic hypotension or somnolence, which can contribute to nocturnal falls.
"On-off" phenomenon	**Goal:** To avoid or minimize unpredictable off periods.
	Actions to take: • **Pharmacological strategies:** Any of the above strategies for "wearing-off" might be helpful initially. Eventually all these actions will fail. It is dangerous to ever withdraw a patient completely from levodopa, especially abruptly, since this may produce an NMS-like syndrome.[12] • **Consider DBS surgery for severe refractory cases.**
Dose failures or "delayed on"	**Goal:** Dose failures may occur idiosyncratically for no apparent reason or due to dietary factors.
	Actions to take: • **Ensure levodopa dosing is at least 1 hour prior to or 2 hours after meals.** • **Reduce the protein content of meals or cluster protein intake to one meal.**
"Super-off"	**Goal:** To quickly reestablish effective voluntary movement and reduce the pain and anxiety that may accompany a "super-off."
	Actions to take: • **Chew immediate-release levodopa.** • **Use a solution of dissolved levodopa:** Levodopa may be dissolved in carbonated water or an ascorbic acid (vitamin C) solution. Caution—may lead to an overuse syndrome. • **Use orally dissolving levodopa.** • **Apomorphine injections:** Very rapid onset of action and very effective in rapidly aborting off states, but has a very short duration of action. • **Add a rotigatine patch to the regimen to avoid abrupt "trough" periods, giving a basal level of stimulation. Good for bridge when patients are perioperatively N.P.O.**[13]

Table 6.2 (Continued)	
TREATMENT OF MOTOR FLUCTUATIONS	
Freezing	**Goal:** Break the motor block, allowing the initiation of movement and decrease the propensity for motor blocks to occur.
	Actions to take:
	• **Add a DA to extend the DTR, which may reduce the frequency of freezing.**
	• **Mechanical stimulation:**
	The patient touching the top of foot with a cane, or companion touching the patient or giving a controlled push, may break a freeze.
	• **Visual cues and other techniques:**
	Angling a cane or a rolling walker with a projected laser line to step over may break the freeze, as may a rhythmic activity such as singing a song.

impair a patient (Table 6.3). Physicians have to avoid two extremes, undertreating a patient, which is easy to do because of a nihilistic acceptance that the patient's neurodegenerative disease is incurable and will cause impairment, or over-treating a patient as an overreaction to complaints by a patient or family member with unrealistic expectations. It is best to change one drug at a time and observe the change for at least three to four weeks. Even at stable doses, Parkinson's disease control varies considerably from day to day in a patient with even moderately advanced disease. Overreacting to a period of response of only a few days is like over-steering a boat, and this impatience will lead to errors. Since it takes four to five half-lives to reach a drug's serum steady-state and then at least another week or two of observation to assess the effects of drug changes, modifications should generally be made no more frequently than every two to four weeks unless intolerable side effects occur. For clarity, some simple steps to consider with each of the potential motor complications are presented below in table format. For advanced patients refractory to medication changes, deep brain stimulation surgery (DBS) may be a consideration if the patient is young and cognitively intact, does not have uncontrolled depression or severe systemic diseases, and has a history of a prior good response to levodopa.

Conclusions

Patients with Parkinson's disease have a somewhat predictable progression of disease, with each stage introducing new therapeutic challenges. Disability, both from disease progression as well as from medication side effects can be anticipated and managed. Simple strategies can be employed in a rational manner once the disabling phenomenology has been correctly identified. At the core of this strategy is having a good understanding of the dopamine replacement therapy options, both levodopa and the dopamine agonists. Each class has advantages and significant side effect profiles that must be appreciated in order to use them properly. Since these benefits and risks vary with the age of the patient and the stage of disease, both thoughtful short-term and long-term

Table 6.3 Treatment Approachs for Managing Dyskinesias

TREATMENT OF DYSKINESIAS

Peak-dose choreiform dyskinesias	**Goal:** Since this is a peak-dose phenomenon in most cases, the general goal is to reduce the peak dose concentration, or C_{max}, of levodopa while maintaining sufficient brain dopamine levels over time to prevent any deterioration into a disabling parkinsonian state.
	Actions to take: • **Do nothing:** Unless the patient's choreiform dyskinesias are disabling, treatment may not be needed. • **Lower the levodopa dose but shorten the dosing interval.** • **Add a low dose of a dopamine agonist and reduce the levodopa dose.** • **Replace levodopa entirely with a dopamine agonist.** • **Add a COMT-I or MAOB-I and reduce the levodopa dose.** • **Add amantadine:** Amantadine has direct anti-dyskinetic effects that may be pronounced.[14,15] • **Consider DBS:** DBS can maintain good "on" state while minimizing dyskinesias.
Afternoon/ evening dyskinesias	**Goal:** Minimize dyskinesias that appear/worsen as the day's doses of levodopa progressively increase the brain's dopamine levels. This is very common with use of controlled-release formulations.
	Actions to take: • **Switch from controlled-release to immediate-release entirely, or use controlled-release formulation only in the early part of the day and then IR levodopa in the afternoon and evening.**
Diphasic dyskinesias	**Goal:** To reduce the dyskinesias that appear both as the brain concentration of dopamine rises following a dose and then falls towards the end of a dose cycle.
	Actions to take: While the above techniques can be used, these dyskinesias are typically refractory and may require DBS surgery to control (please see the Chapter 9 for details).
Dystonic posturing	**Goal:** Since this is usually a low-dose phenomenon, the main goal is to raise DRT high enough to return a patient to a good "on" state.
	Actions to take: • **Do nothing:** Often only minor foot inversion on one side is present. If it does not interfere with walking and is not painful, special actions may not be needed; otherwise, see above under *morning "off" periods*. • **Morning dystonia:** Same; see above under *morning "off" periods*. • **Peak-dose dystonia:** This is much less common and can be identified by the fact that it presents consistently 20–40 minutes following a dose. It can be treated similarly to peak-dose dyskinesias as noted above. Some patients are refractory and when severe may require DBS surgery.

strategies have to be used. In patients with young-onset PD, initial treatment strategies vary and must be individualized to the situation. The core therapy in the aged and advanced stages, though, is levodopa. Adjunctive therapies such as enzyme inhibitors (MAOB-I and COMT-I) and amantadine may also have important roles across the spectrum of disease.

The above recommendations are intended as a guide. As the disease advances, a movement disorder specialist can be an invaluable assistant to the primary neurologist and the primary care provider. Deep brain stimulation surgery has also added a new dimension to the treatment of advancing disease (Chapter 9). Until a cure is found, the intelligent implementation of each of these therapeutic options remains the best hope for maintaining a meaningful functional motor status for our patients.

References

1. Stocchi F. The hypothesis of the genesis of motor complications and continuous dopaminergic stimulation in the treatment of Parkinson's disease. *Parkinsonism Relat Disord.* Jan 2009;15(Suppl 1):S9–S15.

2. Investigators PSGCC. Long-term effect of initiating pramipexole vs. levodopa in early Parkinson's disease. *Arch Neurol.* May 2009;66(5):563–570.

3. Ahlskog JE, Muenter MD. Frequency of levodopa-related dyskinesias and motor fluctuations as estimated from the cumulative literature. *Mov Disord.* May 2001;16(3):448–458.

4. Nutt JG. Motor fluctuations and dyskinesia in Parkinson's disease. *Parkinsonism Relat Disord.* Oct 2001;8(2):101–108.

5. Fahn S, Oakes D, Shoulson I, et al. Levodopa and the progression of Parkinson's disease. *N Engl J Med.* Dec 9 2004;351(24):2498–2508.

6. Kostic V, Przedborski S, Flaster E, Sternic N. Early development of levodopa-induced dyskinesias and response fluctuations in young-onset Parkinson's disease. *Neurol.* Feb 1991;41(2 (Pt 1):202–205.

7. Parkinson's Study Group. Entacapone improves motor fluctuations in levodopa-treated Parkinson's disease patients. Parkinson's Study Group. *Ann Neurol.* Nov 1997;42(5):747–755.

8. Brooks DJ, Sagar H. Entacapone is beneficial in both fluctuating and non-fluctuating patients with Parkinson's disease: a randomised, placebo controlled, double blind, six month study. *J Neurol Neurosurg & Psychiatry.* Aug 2003;74(8):1071–1079.

9. Rascol O, Brooks DJ, Melamed E, et al. Rasagiline as an adjunct to levodopa in patients with Parkinson's disease and motor fluctuations (LARGO, Lasting effect in Adjunct therapy with Rasagiline Given Once daily, study): a randomised, double-blind, parallel-group trial. *Lancet.* Mar 12–18 2005;365(9463):947–954.

10. Golbe LI, Lieberman AN, Muenter MD, et al. Deprenyl in the treatment of symptom fluctuations in advanced Parkinson's disease. *Clin Neuropharmacol.* Feb 1988;11(1):45–55.

11. Parkinson's Study Group. A randomized placebo-controlled trial of rasagiline in levodopa-treated patients with Parkinson's disease and motor fluctuations: the PRESTO study. *Arch Neurol.* Feb 2005;62(2):241–248.

12. Toru M, Matsuda O, Makiguchi K, Sugano K. Neuroleptic malignant syndrome-like state following a withdrawal of anti-parkinsonian drugs. *J Nerv Ment Dis.* May 1981;169(5):324–327.

13. Wullner U, Kassubek J, Odin P, et al. Transdermal rotigotine for the perioperative management of Parkinson's disease. *J Neural Transm.* Jul 2010;117(7):855–859.

14. Crosby NJ, Deane KH, Clarke CE. Amantadine for dyskinesia in Parkinson's disease. *Cochrane Database Syst Rev.* 2003(2):CD003467.

15. Snow BJ, Macdonald L, McAuley D, Wallis W. The effect of amantadine on levodopa-induced dyskinesias in Parkinson's disease: a double-blind, placebo-controlled study. *Clin Neuropharmacol.* Mar–Apr 2000;23(2):82–85.

Chapter 7

Non-Motor Complications in Parkinson's Disease

Barbara S. Connolly and Connie Marras

Parkinson's disease was first recognized by its classical motor symptoms; namely, rest tremor, rigidity, bradykinesia, and postural instability. However, over time it has become increasingly evident that patients with PD may have a wide variety of non-motor symptoms as well. Often unrecognized, and therefore untreated, these symptoms can contribute substantially to the overall quality of life and disease burden of these patients as well as their caregivers. Awareness of these potential symptoms and periodic questioning of patients is the key to recognition and successful management. In this chapter we will review the most common non-motor symptoms (Table 7.1) and address the current available treatment options (Table 7.2 for medications and dosages). Studies of treatment for non-motor PD symptoms are limited in many areas and high-quality evidence may be lacking.

Mood Disorders

Depression

Depression is the most common mood disorder associated with Parkinson's disease, with a prevalence of approximately 35 percent, although higher rates are often seen in later disease stages.[1] Depression can be missed during clinical assessments because otherwise classical signs of depression, such as psychomotor retardation, may be masked or misinterpreted as motoric features of PD, such as poverty of movement and facial masking. Additionally, reduced participation in activities may be attributed to the physical challenges faced by patients.

Traditional antidepressants used in the general population, including selective serotonin reuptake inhibitors (SSRIs), serotonin and norepinephrine reuptake inhibitors (SNRIs), and tricyclic antidepressants (TCAs), are also used for PD patients. The lack of comparative trials makes a choice of a single medication difficult, and there is no current consensus about a preferred medication.[2] SSRIs are the most commonly prescribed class for PD-related depression,[3] and a recent randomized controlled trial (RCT) found both paroxetine (SSRI) and venlafaxine XR (SNRI) to significantly improve depression.[4] The secondary amine TCAs nortriptyline and desipramine are also likely to be efficacious,[2]

Table 7.1 Non-Motor Manifestations of Parkinson's Disease

Mood Disorders	Depression
	Anxiety
	Apathy
Cognitive Impairment	Mild cognitive impairment
	Dementia
Psychotic Symptoms	Illusions
	Hallucinations
	Delusions
Sleep Disturbance	Vivid dreams
	Insomnia
	Excessive daytime sleepiness
	REM sleep behavior disorder
	Restless legs syndrome
	Periodic limb movements of sleep
Fatigue	
Dopamine-Induced Impulsive and Compulsive Disorders	Impulse-control disorders
	Punding
	Dopamine dysregulation syndrome
Autonomic Dysfunction	Orthostatic hypotension
	Hyperhydrosis
	Urinary dysfunction
	Urgency
	Frequency
	Nocturia
	Gastrointestinal disturbance
	Drooling
	Nausea
	Constipation
	Dysphagia
	Sexual Dysfunction
	Loss of libido
	Erectile dysfunction
Sensory Symptoms	Pain
	Paresethesias
	Olfactory dysfunction

but cautious use of this medication class is necessary due to the potential anticholinergic side effects, including cognitive impairment, sleepiness, and hallucinations. Risk of serotonin syndrome is present with concurrent use of a monoamine oxidase-B (MAO-B) inhibitor (selegiline or rasagiline) and some antidepressants (fluoxetine, venlafaxine). For drug-resistant cases, PD-related depression, adjunctive cognitive behavioral therapy or electro-convulsive therapy (ECT) can be tried.

Table 7.2 Medications and Typical Dose Ranges for Pharmacological Management of Non-motor Symptoms

Anxiety or Depression	SSRI, SNRI, TCA typical doses*
Dementia	Rivastigmine 1.5–6mg bid (or transdermal patch)
	Donepezil 5–10mg daily
	Galantamine 4–12mg bid
Hallucinations or Delusions	Quetiapine 12.5–400mg, typically at night, may add smaller morning dose
	Clozapine 6.25–50mg/d (with CBC monitoring)
Excessive Daytime Sleepiness	Methylphenidate 10mg tid
REM Sleep Behavior Disorder	Clonazepam 0.5–2mg qhs
	Melatonin 3–15mg qhs
Restless Legs Syndrome or Periodic Limb Movements of Sleep (PLMS)	Pramipexole 0.25–0.75mg taken 1–3 hours before bedtime
	Ropinirole 0.25–6mg taken 1–3 hours before bedtime
	Rotigotine 1–3mg/24 hours
	Levodopa + carbidopa/benserazide 50–200mg 1–3 hours before bedtime
	Gabapentin 300–1200mg 1–3 hours before bedtime
	Opioids (codeine, oxycodone, methadone)
Additional PLMS Medications	Clonazepam 0.5–2mg before bedtime
	Baclofen 10–30mg before bed
Sialorrhea	Atropine 1% 1–2 drops up to 4 times/day
	Glycopyrrolate 1mg 3 times/day
	Ipratropium bromide 1–2 sprays up to 4 times/day
	Botulinum toxin type A or B injections into salivary glands
Orthostatic Hypotension	Fludrocortisone 0.05–0.2mg/day
	Midodrine 2.5–10mg 3 times/day
Urinary Dysfunction	Oxybutynin 2.5mg bid, increase cautiously to max 5mg 5 times/day
	Tolterodine 2mg bid
Nausea, Anorexia, Vomiting	Domperidone 10mg tid, max 20mg 3–4 times/day if severe
Constipation	General measures, see text
Erectile Dysfunction	Sildenafil 50mg 1 hour before sexual activity, range 25–100mg
	Tadalafil 10–20mg 30 minutes before sexual activity, range 5–20mg

SSRI, selective serotonin reuptake inhibitor; SNRI, serotonin norepinephrine reuptake inhibitor; TCA, tricyclic antidepressant

*Fluoxetine and venlafaxine are contraindicated with concurrent use of a monoamine oxidase-B inhibitor.

Anxiety

Anxiety is more common in female and younger PD patients and often coexists with depression.[5] Generalized anxiety disorder, panic disorder with or without agoraphobia, social phobia, and anxiety without fulfilling DSM criteria for anxiety disorder have all been reported.[6] Anxiety can be a primary diagnosis or may be related to the cycle of dopaminergic treatment; present only when dopaminergic medications are not working optimally ("off"), or when transitioning from "on" to "off." Psychosocial interventions may be beneficial, and modification of dopaminergic therapy may treat "off" anxiety. SSRIs, low-dose TCAs, and buspirone are also used.[7] Although benzodiazepines have well-known anxiolytic properties, they are not typically recommended for PD patients due to the potential adverse effects including cognitive and psychomotor impairment.

Apathy

Apathy refers to negative symptoms such as blunted emotions, loss of interest, lack of motivation, and lack of productivity. It commonly co-occurs with depression and cognitive impairment, and may also herald cognitive decline and dementia in PD.[8,9] Studies on this topic are limited, and treatment is not well-defined, although levodopa may improve "on"-state motivation.[10]

Psychotic Symptoms

Psychotic symptoms in Parkinson's disease consist of illusions, hallucinations, and (usually paranoid) delusions. Well-formed visual hallucinations are most commonly reported, but patients may also experience auditory, tactile, olfactory, somatic, and gustatory hallucinations, a sense of presence (a vision or sensation of something passing), or misidentification syndromes.

Management of psychotic symptoms should begin with confirmation that the patients' symptoms are not due to delirium from non-PD medications or a general medical condition, such as an infection. PD-related psychotic symptoms may be a primary manifestation of the disease itself or a side effect of treatment. Levodopa, dopamine agonists, MAO-B inhibitors, catechol-O-methyl transferase (COMT) inhibitors, anticholinergics, and amantadine can all cause psychotic symptoms. Dose reduction or complete withdrawal of the offending medication(s) may be necessary. Clinicians should balance motor benefit from a particular medication with its likelihood of causing these symptoms. Removal or reduction of medications in the following order is suggested: anticholinergics, amantadine, MAO-B inhibitors, COMT inhibitors, dopamine agonists. Levodopa has the best risk–benefit ratio, and in some cases levodopa monotherapy may be necessary.

Treatment with antipsychotic medications may be complicated by worsening of motor symptoms. Quetiapine and clozapine have the lowest risk of exacerbating parkinsonism. Although there is a lack of evidence for the effectiveness of quetiapine, it is often tried before clozapine, which has clear efficacy, since frequent blood monitoring is required with use of clozapine due to the risk of agranulocytosis.

Cognitive Impairment and Dementia

Cognitive impairment in Parkinson's disease may affect any number of cognitive domains, particularly executive function, psychomotor speed, memory, visuospatial processing, and attention.[11] Mild cognitive impairment (MCI) and PD dementia (PDD) are differentiated by the lack of interference of cognitive impairment in social and occupational functioning in PD-MCI. PD-MCI is seen in 27 percent of all non-demented PD patients,[11] while PDD has a point prevalence of approximately 30 percent[12] and affects up to 80 percent of patients over the course of their disease.[13] PD-MCI is a risk factor for progression to PDD.

Management of cognitive complaints in PD should start with a review of the patient's medication list. Many of the medications used to treat PD can affect cognition, including dopamine agonists, anticholinergics (such as trihexyphenidyl, used for tremor), amantadine, selegiline (MAO-B inhibitor) and entacapone (COMT inhibitor). Discontinuation of these medications can be undertaken in the same manner as described above for psychosis. Medications targeting non-PD symptoms (such as anticholinergics used for bladder dysfunction) can also contribute to decreased memory and attention (Table 7.3) and should be minimized. PD-MCI is not typically treated pharmacologically, although studies in this area are planned. Cholinesterase inhibitors are used for management of PDD. Conclusive evidence exists for rivastigmine, but donepezil and galantamine may also be effective.[2] Memantine is not typically used, due to conflicting evidence for its effectiveness.

Dopamine-Related Impulsive and Compulsive Behaviors

Dopamine-related impulsive and compulsive behaviors comprise impulse-control disorders (ICDs), "punding," and dopamine dysregulation syndrome (DDS). ICDs are a variety of pleasurable behaviors performed to a detrimental level, such as pathological gambling, compulsive shopping or eating, or hypersexual behavior, that occur in approximately 14 percent of PD patients.[14] "Punding" is a term used to describe a complex, superfluous, stereotyped

Table 7.3 Common Non-PD Medications with the Potential to Impair Cognition
Narcotic analgesics
Hypnotics (e.g., benzodiazepines, zopiclone, zaleplon)
Anticholinergics (e.g., TCAs*, tolterodine, oxybutnin, solifenacin)
Antihistamines/decongestants
Corticosteroids
Muscle relaxants (e.g., baclofen, cyclobenzaprine)
*Tricyclic antidepressants

action or utterance, while DDS refers to the compulsive use (typically overuse) of dopaminergic medication occurring in 3–4 percent of patients.[15] All of these behaviors can result in an impairment of personal, social, or occupational functioning.

Since these disorders are related to the use of dopaminergic medications, management typically involves an enforced gradual reduction or elimination of the offending agent. Dopamine agonists are most often the cause of ICDs, while levodopa more frequently causes punding and DDS. When weaning dopamine agonists in cases of ICDs, clinicians should monitor patients for symptoms of dopamine agonist withdrawal syndrome (DAWS), such as anxiety, panic attacks, depression, fatigue, pain, orthostatic hypotension, and drug cravings.[16] DDS can be challenging to treat and generally involves working closely with the patient's pharmacy to prevent the use of multiple prescriptions or early refills.

Sleep-Related Disturbances

Sleep-related disorders are frequently experienced by PD patients. They may be primary to the illness or secondary to medication. Restless legs syndrome (RLS) and periodic limb movements of sleep (PLMS) are more common in PD than in the general population and can result in disrupted sleep. RLS is characterized by a desire to move the limbs, often accompanied by unpleasant sensations, particularly during periods of inactivity and at night, and relieved by movement. RLS can be treated with dopaminergic medication, anticonvulsants (e.g., gabapentin), or opioids, although secondary causes including iron deficiency and renal failure should be ruled out first. PLMS can arise independently from RLS, or the two conditions may co-occur. It typically manifests as repetitive flexion movements of the toes, ankles, knees, and hips, and sometimes the arms as well, with a periodicity of 5–90 seconds. Its management is similar to the management of RLS, although benzodiazepines (e.g., clonazepam) and GABA agonists (e.g., baclofen) are also utilized.

Rapid eye movement (REM) sleep behavioral disorder (RBD) may precede the diagnosis of neurodegenerative disease by many years. RBD, defined as abnormal movements and vocalizations while dreaming, is due to the loss of the paralysis that should occur during REM sleep, and may lead to personal injury and/or disruption or injury of a bed partner. The first-line medication is clonazepam; melatonin is also used.

Excessive daytime somnolence (EDS) is usually multifactorial in etiology: a consequence of the disease process, but also linked to reduced sleep quality secondary to PD and use of dopaminergic medication. Those with EDS related to dopamine agonist use may notice sudden onset of sleep, or "sleep attacks." Driving should be avoided by patients experiencing sleep attacks.

Reduced sleep quality may play a role in EDS. Many patients return to an "off" state during the night and develop pain or have difficulty turning and adjusting bedclothes, thus awakening frequently. Instituting a dose of long-acting levodopa at bedtime or an extra levodopa dose in the middle of the night, when a patient awakens to void, may improve sleep. Vivid dreams and insomnia can also lead to sleep disturbance and may be medication- or disease-related. Vivid dreams can occur with use of dopaminergic medications, while insomnia can be associated with a coexistent depression. Stimulant medications such as modafinil, methylphenidate, and sodium oxybate may be beneficial for EDS in some patients.

Fatigue

Distinct from sleepiness, fatigue is a "feeling of abnormal and overwhelming tiredness and lack of energy, distinct both qualitatively and quantitatively from normal tiredness."[17] The etiology of fatigue in PD is unclear, but around half of PD patients report this potentially disabling symptom. Fatigue has been associated with depression and often presents early in the disease course, worsening over time.[18] Methylphenidate may be useful for PD-related fatigue, and antidepressants can be trialed for patients with concurrent depression.

Autonomic Dysfunction

Involvement of the autonomic nervous system in PD may be manifested by orthostatic hypotension, urinary and gastrointestinal disturbances, and sexual dysfunction. Typically unresponsive to levodopa, management of these conditions in PD reflects that of the general population.

Orthostatic Hypotension

Orthostatic hypotension (OH) may be reported by patients as lightheadedness, dizziness, nausea, ache in head or shoulders, visual disturbance, diaphoresis, and/or loss of consciousness. Although PD is usually the underlying cause, dopaminergic medications often aggravate this symptom, as can advanced age, increased temperatures, and postprandial and post-exercise states.[19] Non-pharmacological options include increasing fluid and salt intake, elevating the head of the bed, and/or use of compression stockings or abdominal binders. Patients should be instructed to make slow, careful changes in position. If these fail, midodrine, fludrocortisones, or less commonly, pyridostigmine, yohimbine, and L-threo-3,4-dihydroxyphenylserine (Droxidopa®) can be used to elevate blood pressure. For patients who develop OH while taking a dopaminergic medication, domperidone, a peripheral dopamine antagonist (not available in the United States), may also be beneficial.

Hyperhidrosis

Sweating dysfunction can cause physical, social, and emotional impairment. Approximately 45 percent of PD patients report excessive sweating, which may occur when a patient is experiencing off periods or dyskinesias, or nocturnally.[18] Management of motor fluctuations, colder room temperatures, cool, comfortable clothing, and increased fluid intake may all improve this symptom.[19]

Urinary Dysfunction

Symptoms of urinary dysfunction in PD consist of urgency, urge incontinence, frequency, and nocturia and typically relate to overactivity of the detrusor muscle of the bladder. Anticholinergic medications, including oxybutynin, tolterodine, and solifenacin, are the mainstay of treatment, although they should be used with caution in individuals with cognitive impairment. Desmopressin has also been utilized for severe nocturia.

Gastrointestinal Symptoms

Drooling, dysphagia, dyspepsia, nausea, gastroparesis, constipation, abdominal pain, and fecal incontinence are all potential gastrointestinal complications of PD. Drooling may be due to autonomic dysfunction but can also be related to dysphagia, reduced swallowing frequency, or even head positioning from a stooped posture. A potentially embarrassing and socially limiting symptom, drooling may be improved with gum-chewing and pharmacologically by local anticholinergic medication such as atropine or glycopyrrolate liquid drops or ipatropium bromide spray, or botulinum toxin injections into the salivary glands.

Dysphagia is more common in the later stages of PD. It may be uncomfortable for patients and can lead to aspiration. Coughing with liquids is the most common manifestation of aspiration. A referral to a speech language pathologist for a swallowing assessment is recommended for suggestions regarding safe swallowing techniques and adjustment of food and liquid textures. Patients and caregivers must be counseled on the relationship of dysphagia with pneumonia. If aspiration is unavoidable with oral intake, a feeding tube may be discussed, but it is not usual therapy.

Nausea is often experienced as an adverse effect of dopaminergic medications, most frequently when therapy is being initiated. Extra carbidopa may reduce this symptom, and domperidone, trimethobenzamide, and ondansetron can be useful. Prochlorperazine and metoclopromide should be avoided due to the risk of worsening parkinsonism.

Constipation is a frequent complaint, which can arise many years before PD is diagnosed. Treatment is the same as in the general population and includes measures such as regular exercise, increasing fluid and fiber intake, avoidance of red meat, stool softeners, bowel stimulants, and suppositories or enemas in severe cases.

Sexual Dysfunction

Loss of libido occurs in about 66 percent of PD patients, while erectile dysfunction is experienced by about 43 percent of males with PD.[20] Depression has been associated with loss of libido, so treatment of this comorbid condition may improve sexual interest. Erectile dysfunction may respond to phosphodiesterase inhibitors or apomorphine.

Sensory Disturbance

Pain, paresthesias, and olfactory dysfunction (anosmia) encompass most sensory symptoms in PD. Pain can be primary or secondary, with musculosketal pain the most common cause. Primary pain may be dysesthetic, burning, radicular or pseudo-radicular, a "heavy feeling," or ill-defined, and is often linked to the "off" phase of motor fluctuations, including commonly early-morning dystonia.[21] Oral (burning mouth syndrome), visceral, and genital pain are also rarely described. In addition to the standard medications for musculoskeletal and neuropathic pain, it is important to elucidate whether the pain is related to the "off" phase, and if so, PD medication adjustments may alleviate these periods. Anosmia has been identified as a prodromal finding in PD, having a high sensitivity but low specificity, since up to one-third of elderly persons have olfactory loss.[22]

Conclusion

PD non-motor symptoms are diverse and can occur at any time along the disease course. These symptoms may have a substantial impact on the quality of life of patients and their caregivers. Awareness of the potential symptoms and recognition of symptoms in PD patients is vital for their successful management. Determining whether a symptom is primary to PD or secondary to PD medication use may guide treatment decisions. For many symptoms, management mimics that of the general population, often with limited or no evidence for effectiveness in PD patients. It is important to remain mindful of medications that may cause cognitive side effects or worsen parkinsonism.

References

1. Van der Hoek TC, Bus BAA, Matui P, van der Marck MA, Esselink RA, Tendolkar I. Prevalence of depression in Parkinson's disease: effects of disease stage, motor subtype and gender. *J Neurol Sci*. 2011;310:220–224.

2. Seppi K, Weintraub D, Coelho M, et al. The Movement Disorder Society evidence-based medicine review update: treatments for the non-motor symptoms of Parkinson's disease. *Mov Disord*. 2011;26(S3):S42–S80.

3. Aarsland D, Pahlhagen S, Ballard CG, Ehrt U, Svenningsson P. Depression in Parkinson's disease—epidemiology, mechanisms and management. *Nat Rev Neurol*. 2012;8(1):35–47.

4. Richard IH, McDermott MP, Kurlan R, et al. A randomized, double-blind, placebo-controlled trial of antidepressants in Parkinson's disease. *Neurology*. 2012;78:1229–1236.

5. Brown RG, Landau S, Hindle JV, et al. Depression and anxiety related subtypes in Parkinson's disease. *JNNP*. 2011;82:803–809.

6. Bolluk B, Ozel-Kizil ET, Akbostanci MC, Atbasglu EC. Social anxiety in patients with Parkinson's disease. *J Neuropsychiatry Clin Neurosci*. 2010;22(4):390–394.

7. Tan LCS. Mood disorders in Parkinson's disease. *Parkinson Relat Disord*. 2012;18(Suppl 1);S74–S76.

8. Starkstein S, Merello M, Jorge R, Brockman S, Bruce D, Power B. The syndromal validity and nosological position of apathy in Parkinson's disease. *Mov Disord*. 2009;15:1211–1216.

9. Dujardin K, Sockeel P, Delliaux M, Destee A, Defebvre I. Apathy may herald cognitive decline and dementia in PD. *Mov Disord*. 2009;24:2391–2397.

10. Czernecki V, Pillon B, Houeto JL, Pochon JB, Dubois B. Motivation, reward, and Parkinson's disease: influence of dopatherapy. *Neuropsychologia*. 2002;40(13):2257–2267.

11. Litvan I, Aarsland D, Adler CH, et al. MDS task force on mild cognitive impairment in Parkinson's disease: critical review of PD-MCI. *Mov. Disord.* 2011;26(10):1814–1824.

12. Aarsland D, Zaccai J, Brayne C. A systematic review of prevalence studies of dementia in Parkinson's disease. *Mov Disord.* 2005;20:1255–1263.

13. Aarsland D, Andersen K, Larsen JP, Lolk A, Kragh-Sørensen P. Prevalence and characteristics of dementia in Parkinson's disease: an 8-year prospective study. *Arch Neurol.* 2003;60:387–392.

14. Weintraub D, Koester J, Potenza MN, et al. Impulse control disorders in Parkinson's disease: a cross-sectional study of 3090 patients. *Arch Neurol.* 2010;67(5):589–595.

15. O'Sullivan SS, Evans AH, Lees AJ. Dopamine dysregulation syndrome. An overview of its epidemiology, mechanisms, and management.*CNS Drugs.* 2009;23(2):157–170.

16. Rabinak CA, Nirenberg MJ. Dopamine agonist withdrawal syndrome in Parkinson's disease. *Arch Neurol.* 2010;67:58–63.

17. Brown RG, Dittner A, Findley L, Wessley SC. The Parkinson's fatigue scale. *Parkinsonism Relat Disord.* 2005;11:49–55.

18. Friedman JH, Brown RG, Comella C, et al. Fatigue in Parkinson's disease: a review. *Mov Disord.* 2007;22(3):297–308.

19. Bernal-Pacheco O, Limotai N, Go, CL, Fernandez HH. Nonmotor manifestations in Parkinson's disease. *Neurologist.* 2012;18(1):1–16.

20. Kummer A, Cardoso F, Teixeira AL. Loss of libido in Parkinson's disease. *J Sex Med.* 2009;6(4):1024–1031.

21. Giuffrida R, Vingerhoets FJ, Bogousslavsky J, Ghika J. [Pain in Parkinson's disease]. *Rev Neurol (Paris).* 2005;161(4):407–418.

22. Postuma RB, Aarsland D, Barone P, et al. Identifying prodromal Parkinson's disease: pre-motor disorders in Parkinson's disease. *Mov Disord.* 2012;27(5):617–626.

Chapter 8

The Follow-Up Visit for Parkinson's Disease

Stephen G. Reich

The insidious progression of Parkinson's disease, with relatively little objective change between outpatient visits, belies the fact that it is actually a very dynamic disease with a complex array of motor and non-motor features. Furthermore, the many pharmacological and non-pharmacological options available to treat PD, and the need to "fine-tune" and balance carefully the beneficial and deleterious effects of medications, add to the challenge, as well as the rewards, of managing PD.

The goals for a PD clinic visit are to (1) reevaluate the accuracy of the diagnosis; (2) determine if there has been a change sufficient to necessitate a medication adjustment; (3) screen for problematic medication side effects; (4) assess non-motor aspects of PD; and (5) educate the patient and family. In preparation for a clinic visit, I encourage patients to bring a list of all their medications and the times when taken, as well as a brief list of the issues they would like to discuss. It easy to get overwhelmed with multiple complaints, and when this happens it is helpful to prioritize by asking, "What's the biggest problem you're having now with PD?" Throughout the course of PD, communication between the patient, their family, and the healthcare providers is the key to effective management.

Is It Still Parkinson's Disease?

Approximately 20 percent of patients diagnosed with PD will prove to have an alternative diagnosis at autopsy—typically a parkinsonian syndrome such as multiple system atrophy (MSA) or progressive supranuclear palsy (PSP).[1] The key to making this distinction during life is being familiar with and looking for "red flags" that cast doubt on the diagnosis of PD.[2] Some of these are obvious at presentation, such as early falls or dementia, both of which happen *late* in the course of PD, but many of the signs suggesting atypical parkinsonism (rather than PD) emerge only over time, requiring reconsideration of the initial diagnosis of PD at each outpatient visit. In addition to early falls and dementia, additional red flags include early hallucinations, early dysautonomia, and early dysphagia. A robust response to levodopa is expected with PD, and failure to respond should call into doubt the diagnosis (the exception is that the rest tremor may not be very levodopa-responsive).

While a full discussion of the red flags casting doubt on the diagnosis of PD and the characteristics of each parkinsonian syndrome, is beyond the scope of this chapter, some key findings include slowing or restriction of vertical eye movements (suggesting PSP), anterocollis or retrocollis, suggesting MSA or PSP respectively, rapid progression, apraxia, aphasia, spasticity, or cerebellar signs (see also Chapter 3). The most reassuring signs that PD is the correct diagnosis include a typical resting tremor, unilateral or asymmetrical onset of signs, beneficial and sustained response to levodopa with the eventual appearance of fluctuations and dyskinesias, and the absence of red flags. Aside from a brief survey for atypical signs (red flags) and unrelated problems, most patients with PD require only a brief examination during a follow-up visit, and it more useful to spend the majority of the time discussing symptoms and functioning.

Is a Medication Change Needed?

As most people with PD report some progression, even if minimal, between visits, there is a temptation to respond with an increase in medication. The key is to determine which changes necessitate a medication adjustment and which do not. This starts by educating patients that the goal in treating PD is not to alleviate all of the symptoms and signs, but instead, to use the least amount of medication that controls symptoms to an "acceptable" degree and allows the person to function at an "acceptable" level. Of course, what is "acceptable" varies from person to person, emphasizing that the treatment of PD must be *individualized*.

With some exceptions, there are three reasons to make a medication change during a follow-up visit. First, if there are significant medication side effects. Second, if there are *problematic* levodopa-related motor fluctuations, notably "off" time or dyskinesias. Mild fluctuations and dyskinesias are usually well tolerated. This is particularly the case with dyskinesias that often bother the family more than the patient, and in that circumstance, the appropriate treatment is education and reassurance. The third reason for a medication change is when the patient is no longer functioning at an acceptable level. Patients should be educated from the first visit that the most important barometer to assess the severity of PD is how much it interferes with their normal personal and professional functioning. So, even if there has been some progression of symptoms since the last visit, if they have not translated into a meaningful decline in functioning, then a medication change is usually not necessary.

There are several other points about medication management that need consideration during outpatient visits. Be sure to determine the times of day when patients take their medication, particularly levodopa. If not counseled otherwise, patients may space it out over the course of the entire day, meaning that the last dose is at bedtime. Most people with PD do not need levodopa near bedtime, unless PD symptoms interfere with sleep. Instead, levodopa should be taken during the waking/active day, usually at four-hour intervals.

Another issue is polypharmacy. Because most PD patients are eventually on several medications, it is important to assess critically whether a medication is helping. To determine which drugs are helping, it is important to eliminate only one medication at a time, and to do so gradually. Similarly, when initiating medication, start with a low dose, especially in the elderly, and escalate gradually. Patients should be educated about side effects, realistic expectations, and that it may take a while to reach a therapeutic dose, particularly for an agonist. Ideally, only one drug should be started or stopped at a time. I emphasize to patients that initial side effects often diminish with time and that treatment of PD is largely a matter of "trial and error," again, underscoring the need to individualize therapy. Finally, it is best to write out changes in medication for the patient—what you think you explained clearly, and what seemed to be understood at the visit, may not be so clear to the patient the next day.

Medication Side Effects

Outpatient visits should include a screen for problematic medication side effects. Yet, if patients are educated properly about which side effects to be on guard for, then most of these can be dealt with as they arise, between visits. Furthermore, it is important for patients to understand that, when it comes to treating PD, there is "no free lunch," meaning that most medication side effects are mild and relatively well tolerated compared to their benefit. Examples include mild ankle edema from dopamine agonists; livedo reticularis from amantadine; bright yellow urine from entacapone, and levodopa-induced dyskinesias. A complete review of all potential side effects of anti-PD drugs is not feasible here and only some of the most problematic will be presented; this discussion will not include levodopa-related motor fluctuations (Chapter 6).

Medication-induced somnolence is common in PD, especially with dopamine agonists, and each visit should include an inquiry about sleep—both the quality of nighttime sleep (see next section) and whether there is daytime somnolence; the latter puts the patient at risk for falling asleep behind the wheel. Another important medication side effect is an impulse-control disorder.[3] Recently recognized, this complication can occur with any dopaminergic therapy but more commonly with an agonist. It takes various forms, including pathological gambling, hypersexuality, compulsive shopping, binge eating, and compulsively pursuing hobbies. It is important to warn patients and their family of this potential complication when prescribing. Since these compulsions often take place surreptitiously, they can be challenging to diagnose, and inquiry should be made in a non-judgemental fashion.

Up to 25 percent of PD patients experience hallucinations and delusions, typically in more advanced stages when there is co-morbid cognitive impairment or dementia. Some patients will voluntarily report hallucinations, but others are reticent to do so. I approach this as follows: "Sometimes the medications can play a trick on your mind, causing you to see something that isn't there or have an unusual thought...have you experienced anything like this?" When hallucinations are infrequent, with preserved insight, no intervention is needed, but when they are problematic, then the first step, aside from education and reassurance, is to reduce or eliminate medication (typically starting with everything except levodopa); and when this is not feasible or helpful, then consider prescribing an atypical antipsychotic. The key to managing hallucinations, delusions, and other side effects of anti-PD drugs is being familiar with them, anticipating them, warning the patient and family about them, and querying the patient and spouse each visit. It is said jokingly that the two times someone with PD can be helped the most is when medications are started and when they are stopped—experience with PD has taught that this is not a joke.

Non-Motor Features of PD

Although PD is defined by the classic motor signs of bradykinesia, rest tremor, cogwheel rigidity, and postural instability, it is often the non-motor features of PD that are most problematic for patients and caregivers. Yet, despite being significant sources of disability and impacting negatively on patients' quality of life, non-motor symptoms are often given inadequate attention. A complete discussion of the non-motor features of PD is beyond the scope of this chapter (see Chapter 7); instead, only selected symptoms will be discussed.[4] The non-motor symptoms of PD can be divided into the following categories: *sensory*; *autonomic*; *sleep*; and *neuropsychiatric*. Appreciate that non-motor PD symptoms can fluctuate with the timing of levodopa, just like motor symptoms and signs.

Sensory symptoms of PD include akathisia (an inner sense of restlessness), which overlaps with a common symptom voiced by patients: an "inner" or subjective tremor. Decreased sense of smell is common in PD and may precede motor signs. There may be pain in PD. Fatigue is probably the most common and often the most debilitating sensory symptom of PD. It may be due to a sleep disorder, general medical problem, or deconditioning, but in most cases, a specific cause other than PD itself is not found.

Autonomic problems are both an intrinsic part of PD and a complication of its treatment. Sexual dysfunction, in both men and women, is common but infrequently discussed by patients and inadequately assessed by healthcare professionals. Orthostatic hypotension is common in PD, and in addition to presenting with typical near-syncope, it can also cause fatigue, poor concentration, and pain across the shoulders when standing. Furthermore, orthostatic hypotension may be asymptomatic, making the patient at risk when a medication is increased or added. Drenching sweats are part of PD, often at night, and they may fluctuate with levodopa.

Sleep problems are nearly universal in PD. The motor symptoms of PD (as well as leg cramps) may interfere with initiating or maintaining sleep, such as tremor at bedtime, trouble turning in bed or getting comfortable in bed. Depression and anxiety can cause insomnia. Restless legs syndrome appears to occur more commonly in PD. Many patients with PD have a REM sleep behavioral disorder, and it is now also appreciated that this is often a precursor to PD. This is rarely brought up by the patient unless they are aware of vivid dreams or if they have jumped out of bed in the process of enacting a dream. Instead, it is the caregiver who relates that the patient often talks, yells, and physically enacts dreams, which can involve grabbing or hitting the bed partner. Daytime sleepiness is very common in PD and is usually due to inadequate nighttime sleep. Additionally, many of the drugs used to treat PD, particularly dopamine agonists, cause somnolence.

The final category of non-motor symptoms in PD is neuropsychiatric, some of which have already been discussed including hallucinations and delusions. Anxiety and depression, occurring together or separately, are common in PD, and should be screened for at each visit. Both respond to standard therapies, and when they are severe, a psychiatrist should be involved. Many patients with PD eventually develop dementia but before that point often experience milder forms of cognitive impairment, particularly executive dysfunction.[5] In additional to historical information each visit, in our clinic we also perform an annual Montreal Cognitive Assessment as a screen for cognitive decline. When there is cognitive impairment or dementia, it is important to screen for treatable causes and critically evaluate all PD and non-PD medications, especially those with anticholinergic activity.

Educating the Patient and Family

One of the most important "therapies" in the management of PD is education. In addition to screening motor and non-motor symptoms and functioning, educating patients is an equally important objective each visit. Ultimately, successful management of a chronic illness such as PD goes beyond just medication and requires patients and care partners to be students of their disease. Education begins at the first visit, by explaining how the diagnosis is made, emphasizing that the progression is slow, that effective therapies are available, and the need to focus on the "big picture" of functioning and less on individual symptoms and signs. When medications are started, patients and their care partners should be clear on the goals of treatment as well as potential side effects.

The more knowledgeable the patient and care partner are about PD, the easier it is to have a cooperative doctor–patient relationship. Support groups can be very helpful, but for the newly diagnosed, encountering people in more advanced stages of PD can be frightening. Similarly, when reading about PD, patients should be forewarned about picking up only on "worst-case scenarios." Despite the importance of patient education, appreciate that patients and their care partners may not be as eager, especially early on, to learn as you are to teach about PD, which again emphasizes the need to individualize therapy and adhere to Osler's maxim that "it is more important to know the person the disease has than the disease the person has."

Education is also an effective means to boost morale and encourage hope by emphasizing research progress and encouraging participation in clinical trials. In this same vein, clinic visits are also an opportunity to screen for and emphasize the positive to patients and their care partners, and when appropriate, compliment them on their perseverance. One of the most important questions to ask of the care partner each visit is "How are you holding up?" This not only opens the door to assessing their needs but also lets them know that their efforts and concerns are recognized.

References

1. Hughes AJ, Daniel SE, Kilford L, Lees AJ. Parkinson's disease: a clinico-pathological study of 100 cases. *J Neurol Neurosurg Psychiatry*. 1992;55:181–184.

2. Köllensperger M, Geser F, Seppi K, et al. Red flags for multiple system atrophy. *Mov Disord*. 2008;23:1093–1099.

3. Weintraub D, Nirenberg MJ. Impulse control and related disorders in Parkinson's disease. *Neurodegener Dis*. 2013;11:63–71.

4. Chaudhuri KR, Healy DG, Schapira AH. Non-motor symptoms of Parkinson's disease: diagnosis and management. *Lancet Neurol*. 2006;5:235–245.

5. Docherty MJ, Burn DJ. Parkinson's disease dementia. *Curr Neurol Neurosci Rep*. 2010;10:292–298.

Chapter 9

When to Consider Deep Brain Stimulation Surgery, and How to Approach It

Kevin R. Cannard

The management of advancing Parkinson's disease has been dramatically changed since the introduction of deep brain stimulation (DBS) surgery in 1987. Its efficacy and safety have been demonstrated in numerous controlled trials[1-6]; these effects are sustained over time[5,7-9] and are superior to those from medication alone.[1,8] The key to employing this treatment option effectively is to understand what the treatment achieves, who is most likely to benefit, when in the course of the disease to use it, and what the risks are when implanting and using DBS.

DBS: An Overview

The DBS system is a permanent, surgically implanted system with three main components: an implanted pulse generator (IPG) that is sometimes called a "neurostimulator" or "battery," a stimulation electrode lead implanted into the brain target, and a lead extension that connects the two (Figure 9.1). Despite its proven clinical efficacy, the exact mechanism by which DBS produces clinical benefit is unclear. The most popular hypothesis is that stimulation, like older ablative lesioning techniques (e.g., pallidotomy), interrupts abnormal signaling in the brain's movement programming loop.[10] This "jamming" of a bad motor signal is a useful hypothesis to share with patients since it easy to understand.

DBS Surgery

Typically a patient is admitted the night before surgery, at which time all PD medications are withheld. During the first phase, the central lead is implanted into a target (typically the subthalamic nucleus or the globus pallidus interna) using highly precise stereotactic surgical techniques while the patient is awake to allow for intraoperative examination. The second phase of surgery is done under general anesthesia. The extension is tunneled underneath the scalp's skin from the lead's proximal end anchored to the external surface of the skull to the IPG (neurostimulator), which is implanted subcutaneously, most commonly

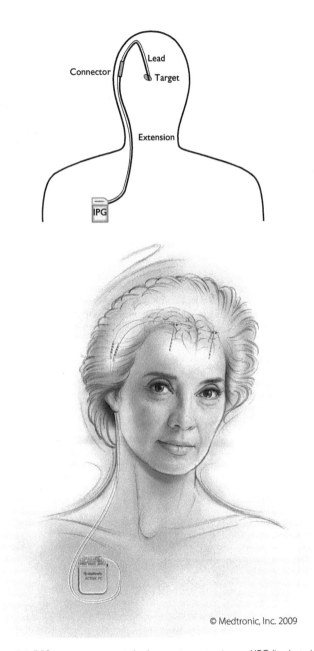

© Medtronic, Inc. 2009

Figure 9.1 DBS system components: lead, connector, extension, and IPG (implanted pulse generator).

in the subclavicular region. Hospitalization typically takes two to four days. The initial programming is delayed two to four weeks and then is refined over a period of weeks to months (see below). Most IPGs last 1.5–4 years, depending partly on the settings and model used, but replacement surgery is a simple outpatient surgery procedure that is often performed under local anesthesia.

Who May Benefit from DBS Surgery and How May It Help Them?

DBS can improve the cardinal motor features of PD (rigidity, bradykinesia, tremor), decrease "off" time, increase "on" time, reduce medication-related motor fluctuations, reduce PD-associated dykinesias and dystonia; and it typically allows the reduction of medications. While DBS provides little improvement in the quality of motor functioning over a patient's best "on" time, it increases the quantity of time spent in that "on" state and reduces the time in the "off" state. The percentage of the day an advanced patient spends in a good "on" time with increased mobility without involuntary movements increases from roughly 25 percent to nearly 65–75 percent, depending on the target used.[11] Rigidity and tremor improve on the order of 50–75 percent, and akinesia improves by 50 percent.[5] Overall, "off" time and "off" motor scores (UPDRS-3) are decreased by half,[5] smoothing out a patient's response to therapy. Patients may no longer experience the intense motor fluctuations such as end-of-dose wearing off, the on-off phenomenon, or dose failures. Evidence for these effects has been demonstrated in numerous, evidence-based and blinded trials.[3,5,11] The motor effects of DBS commonly allow a reduction of dopamine replacement therapy (DRT: levodopa and dopamine agonists) medication by 30–70 percent.[3,12] A good way to set reasonable expectations is to tell patients that the goal of DBS surgery is to substantially increase the time spent in a good "on" state while reducing "off" time. The quality of their "on" states, however, may not change substantially over their presurgical peak motor performance. Quality of life measurements have demonstrated substantial improvement.[13–15]

The greatest value of DBS, thus, is in the reduction of "off" time and the management of the motor fluctuations that come with advancing disease. DBS is a therapy best suited for the intermediate stages of PD, typically when the patient is no longer responding optimally to DRT due to motor fluctuations and dyskinesias. It is not appropriate as an initial therapy, nor is it likely to benefit the very advanced patient enough as to justify the risks.[16] In determining who may benefit, the single most important criteria for DBS surgery selection is that the patient *must* have PD that is clearly *levodopa-responsive*. Other parkinsonian syndromes that are largely unresponsive to levodopa, such as multiple system atrophy, progressive supranuclear palsy, and vascular parkinsonism, will have no response to DBS and must be excluded. Essential tremor can respond to DBS but requires a different target in the brain.

Not all features of PD are improved with DBS. In general, the midline, axial symptoms do not improve much. Gait may have no improvement or only limited benefit. When gait is limited primarily because of prominent bradykinesia and rigidity, it may improve as these features are reduced. Potential gait improvement from DBS is best predicted by gait improvement during peak levodopa "on" time. However, when gait is impaired primarily due to balance problems, postural stability, and freezing (abrupt cessation of movement), significant improvement is unlikely. Since falling and freezing may be the most disabling aspect of a patient's disease, this limitation of DBS should be emphasized to the patient and weighed when considering whether a patient may attain meaningful benefit following surgery. Other features that are not improved include speech, swallowing, autonomic function, mood, and cognition.[12] Speech may even deteriorate.[5,6]

The Ideal Candidate for DBS Surgery

The ideal DBS patient is relatively young (under 70–75), has been treated for 5–10 years with a clear response to levodopa, has developed motor fluctuations that compromise functioning, may spend a significant portion of the day in an "off" state, does not have severe comorbid medical conditions, is cognitively intact, and does not suffer from poorly controlled depression or anxiety.[10,16–18] The degree of benefit is clearly more pronounced in younger patients.[16] Subtle cognitive impairment is frequently present in patients with advancing PD, and this is not disqualifying, but frank dementia is a contraindication to surgery. Formal neuropsychometric testing should be performed on most patients. A formal psychiatric evaluation is strongly recommended, particularly for anyone who has been diagnosed or treated for depression or anxiety. These screening steps will typically be ordered by a movement disorder neurologist who is part of the DBS team. This team may also include neurosurgeons, psychiatrists, neuropsychologist, and therapists. A common selection error is to wait until the patient is too advanced to receive full benefit from the surgery.

Complications

Complications related to DBS may occur during surgery, in the postoperative period, or during the lifetime of the system, and have recently been reviewed across the published literature.[19] Only the most frequent or serious complications are discussed here. These complications arise largely from adverse effects related to the surgical procedure, unwanted effects of stimulation, and malfunction of or infections arising from the system hardware. The most immediate intraoperative complication of concern is intracranial hemorrhage. Hemorrhage is uncommon, occurring 0.6–5.0 percent of surgeries, depending on the center,[19] with older studies tending to have higher rates,[3,11,20] and is seen mainly in patients with a history of hypertension. Most experienced centers now have decreased their rates to around 1 percent[21,22] using newer techniques.[21,22] Hemorrhages are typically small in volume, with the majority leaving no persistent deficits. Postoperatively, some patients have a brief period of confusion following surgery, but this is uncommon and seen primarily in the older patient. Infections more commonly cause some of the most serious complications of DBS treatment, with most centers reporting a rate of 1.5–9.0 percent.[23–25] Wound or scar erosion may occur and produce infections. Most of these are superficial, arising from breaks in the skin. Any exposure of hardware should prompt immediate evaluation. Treatment may require the removal and replacement of hardware and a course of intravenous antibiotics. One of the most vexing complications of surgery is suboptimal placement of the electrode lead tip. This can only be corrected with a second surgery. Some of the adverse effects arise from stimulation of unintended nearby structures. Changes in the array or DBS parameters may resolve this. Transient paresthesias are commonly observed when the amplitude of stimulation is increased. Other amplitude-dependent stimulation side effects can include: dizziness, dystonic posturing of the face or a limb, dysarthria, diplopia, dysphoric states, or double vision. Each of these effects may help the programmer determine where the electrode contact is placed and refine the stimulation parameters. See Table 9.1 for a more complete list of complications.

Programming and Follow-up

After implantation, the DBS system must be programmed, usually beginning 2–4 weeks following surgery. This delay allows for resolution of minor edema around the lead tip that may produce a transient beneficial effect (sometimes called a "micro-lesion effect"). Additional sessions typically take place at intervals of 2–8 weeks by the DBS team. This allows for thousands of different combinations of parameters (Figure 9.6). One of the greatest challenges of DBS therapy is determining the optimal settings for a particular patient. This varies from patient to patient, primarily depending on how closely one of the electrodes is implanted to the intended target (which is quite small) and how close that electrode is to nearby structures that would give rise to adverse effects. Typically, optimization of programming occurs over several sessions that take place over a period of weeks to months. An experienced programmer is needed for this phase. Once an optimal setting has been found, patients will typically need follow-up with the DBS team about every six months. It is important that between those visits the patient continue to be followed by a primary

Table 9.1 Complications
• Surgical Complications
• Intracranial hemorrhage
• Mistargeting of lead into incorrect area
• Seizure
• Unwanted Effects of Stimulation
• Paresthesias: often transient and/or amplitude dependent
• Involuntary contractions/dystonia: often from spread to the internal capsule
• Diplopia
• Dysarthria and/or dysphagia
• Dysphoria/depression/anxiety
• Confusion/cognitive impairment
• Ataxia
• System Hardware Complications
• Device failure: initial, or "battery" wears out
• Lead or extension fracture
• Lead migration from target area
• Lead, lead extension, or IPG erosion through the skin
• Infection: hardware as a nidus or as a pathway via erosion

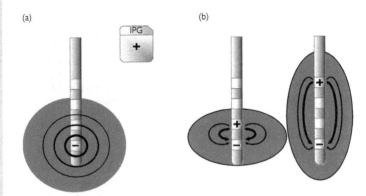

Figure 9.2 DBS lead arrays and stimulation fields. A monopolar array (a) produces a spherical field emanating from a negative lead electrode. This field extends outward to the positive case, which is essentially at an infinite distance. Bipolar arrays (b) use two electrodes of opposite polarity, producing a much tighter field resembling a squashed or elongated sphere. Even more complex fields can be constructed setting two or more electrodes to the same polarity.

neurologist and/or a primary care physician. It is typically recommended that PD medications should be reduced no more than 25 percent initially. Further reductions may be possible later. Physicians should also watch for postoperative depression, which may occur in the weeks or months following surgery. Despite extensive counseling prior to surgery that DBS is not a cure, many patients have unrealistic expectations. Dramatic cases featured on news clips or television shows often contribute to these unrealistic expectations. Prior to

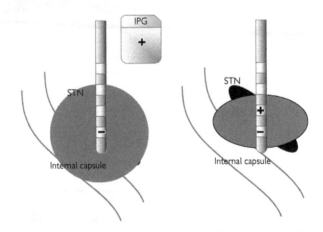

Figure 9.3 DBS lead implanted into a target. The shape of the subthalamic nucleus (STN) is used to illustrate the extension of the stimulation field beyond the borders of the nucleus to the adjacent internal capsule, where it may stimulate the corticospinal tract and cause dystonic posturing. The smaller fields created by bipolar arrays may be helpful in constraining the area of stimulation to avoid unwanted spread.

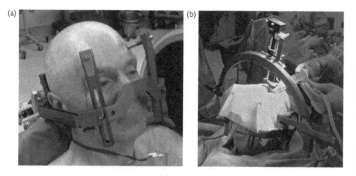

Figure 9.4 A patient with a DBS stereotactic frame placed (a) and later intraoperatively with the arc system secured to the frame (b). The lead holder assembly stage and drive (arrow) holds a cannula through which the DBS lead is inserted into the brain. The stage and drive control the depth of insertion, and may be used for either the microelectrode during brain mapping along a planned pathway or for final placement of the lead being implanted. The stage can be adjusted along the arc and the arc can be tilted/rotated forward or backward, allowing a precise target and pathway to the target to be selected.

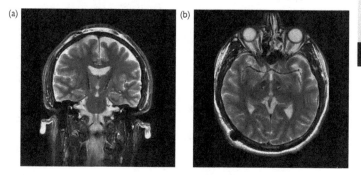

Figure 9.5 DBS leads implanted into bilateral subthalamic nuclei (STN). The leads image as a dark fallout of signal and can be seen extending from just lateral of the ventricles diagonally down to the STN. The more cephlad portions of the leads are out of the plane of the image, and their extension to and through the skull is not seen in this image. The arrows point to the lead tip implanted in the lower edge of the left STN.

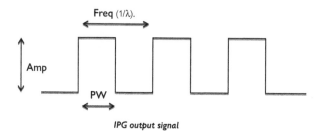

IPG output signal

Figure 9.6 Pulse signal generated by the Implanted Pulse Generator (IPG). Parameters of the stimulation signal that can be adjusted via programming include the amplitude (Amp), the pulse width (PW), and the rate or frequency (Freq), which is just the inverse of the wavelength (λ).

electing to undergo the procedure, it is often helpful to have the patient speak with someone who has undergone DBS surgery.

Conclusion

DBS can be a very powerful and effective treatment for PD. For moderately advanced PD patients, multiple studies have revealed that this therapy in combination with medication is superior to medication alone. In order for it to be employed effectively, patients must be selected carefully. Most importantly, patients must have PD that is clearly levodopa-responsive but compromised by motor fluctuations or dyskinesias incompletely controlled by optimal medication use. Additionally, they must not suffer from dementia or poorly controlled psychiatric disorders. The surgery must be performed by an experienced DBS team, and follow-up should be done in parallel with a neurologist experienced in DBS programming.

References

1. Williams A, Gill S, Varma T, et al. Deep brain stimulation plus best medical therapy versus best medical therapy alone for advanced Parkinson's disease (PD SURG trial): a randomised, open-label trial. *Lancet Neurol.* Jun 2010;9(6):581–591.

2. Burchiel KJ, Anderson VC, Favre J, Hammerstad JP. Comparison of pallidal and subthalamic nucleus deep brain stimulation for advanced Parkinson's disease: results of a randomized, blinded pilot study. *Neurosurgery.* Dec 1999;45(6):1375–1382; discussion 1382–1374.

3. Deuschl G, Schade-Brittinger C, Krack P, et al. A randomized trial of deep-brain stimulation for Parkinson's disease. *N Engl J Med.* Aug 31 2006;355(9):896–908.

4. Hariz MI, Rehncrona S, Quinn NP, Speelman JD, Wensing C. Multicenter study on deep brain stimulation in Parkinson's disease: an independent assessment of reported adverse events at 4 years. *Mov Disord.* Feb 15 2008;23(3):416–421.

5. Krack P, Batir A, Van Blercom N, et al. Five-year follow-up of bilateral stimulation of the subthalamic nucleus in advanced Parkinson's disease. *N Engl J Med.* Nov 13 2003;349(20):1925–1934.

6. Rodriguez-Oroz MC, Obeso JA, Lang AE, et al. Bilateral deep brain stimulation in Parkinson's disease: a multicentre study with 4 years follow-up. *Brain.* Oct 2005;128(Pt 10):2240–2249.

7. Kleiner-Fisman G, Fisman DN, Sime E, Saint-Cyr JA, Lozano AM, Lang AE. Long-term follow up of bilateral deep brain stimulation of the subthalamic nucleus in patients with advanced Parkinson's disease. *J Neurosurg.* Sep 2003;99(3):489–495.

8. Weaver FM, Follett K, Stern M, et al. Bilateral deep brain stimulation vs best medical therapy for patients with advanced Parkinson's disease: a randomized controlled trial. *JAMA.* Jan 7 2009;301(1):63–73.

9. Gervais-Bernard H, Xie-Brustolin J, Mertens P, et al. Bilateral subthalamic nucleus stimulation in advanced Parkinson's disease: five year follow-up. *J Neurol.* Feb 2009;256(2):225–233.

10. Ponce FA, Lozano AM. Deep brain stimulation state of the art and novel stimulation targets. *Prog Brain Res.* 2010;184:311–324.

11. Deep-brain stimulation of the subthalamic nucleus or the pars interna of the globus pallidus in Parkinson's disease. *N Engl J Med.* Sep 27 2001;345(13):956–963.

12. Kleiner-Fisman G, Herzog J, Fisman DN, et al. Subthalamic nucleus deep brain stimulation: summary and meta-analysis of outcomes. *Mov Disord.* Jun 2006;21 Suppl 14:S290–304.

13. Lyons KE, Pahwa R. Long-term benefits in quality of life provided by bilateral subthalamic stimulation in patients with Parkinson's disease. *J Neurosurg.* Aug 2005;103(2):252–255.

14. Diamond A, Jankovic J. The effect of deep brain stimulation on quality of life in movement disorders. *J Neurol Neurosurg Psychiatry.* Sep 2005;76(9):1188–1193.

15. Lezcano E, Gomez-Esteban JC, Zarranz JJ, et al. Improvement in quality of life in patients with advanced Parkinson's disease following bilateral deep-brain stimulation in subthalamic nucleus. *Eur J Neurol.* Jul 2004;11(7):451–454.

16. Derost PP, Ouchchane L, Morand D, et al. Is DBS-STN appropriate to treat severe Parkinson's disease in an elderly population? *Neurology.* Apr 24 2007;68(17):1345–1355.

17. Charles PD, Van Blercom N, Krack P, et al. Predictors of effective bilateral subthalamic nucleus stimulation for PD. *Neurology.* Sep 24 2002;59(6):932–934.

18. Welter ML, Houeto JL, Tezenas du Montcel S, et al. Clinical predictive factors of subthalamic stimulation in Parkinson's disease. *Brain.* Mar 2002;125(Pt 3):575–583.

19. Morishita T, Foote KD, Burdick AP, et al. Identification and management of deep brain stimulation intra- and postoperative urgencies and emergencies. *Parkinsonism Relat Disord.* Mar 2010;16(3):153–162.

20. Voges J, Hilker R, Botzel K, et al. Thirty days complication rate following surgery performed for deep-brain-stimulation. *Mov Disord.* Jul 30 2007;22(10):1486–1489.

21. Sansur CA, Frysinger RC, Pouratian N, et al. Incidence of symptomatic hemorrhage after stereotactic electrode placement. *J Neurosurg.* Nov 2007;107(5):998–1003.

22. Zrinzo L, Foltynie T, Limousin P, Hariz MI. Reducing hemorrhagic complications in functional neurosurgery: a large case series and systematic literature review. *J Neurosurg.* Jan 2012;116(1):84–94.

23. Fenoy AJ, Simpson RK, Jr. Management of device-related wound complications in deep brain stimulation surgery. *J Neurosurg.* Jun 2012;116(6):1324–1332.

24. Sillay KA, Larson PS, Starr PA. Deep brain stimulator hardware-related infections: incidence and management in a large series. *Neurosurgery.* Feb 2008;62(2):360–366; discussion 366–367.

25. Baizabal Carvallo JF, Simpson R, Jankovic J. Diagnosis and treatment of complications related to deep brain stimulation hardware. *Mov Disord.* Jul 2011;26(8):1398–1406.

Chapter 10

Common Challenges and Complications in the Inpatient Setting

Michael J. Soileau and Kelvin L. Chou

Parkinson's disease patients often complain of the care they receive in the inpatient setting. There may be many reasons for their dissatisfaction, but one of the most common is lack of knowledge of or experience with PD symptoms among inpatient providers. Patients with PD are typically responsive to dopaminergic medications and thus do not often need to be hospitalized for their PD, especially in the early to moderate stages. As they advance, they may develop motor fluctuations and dyskinesias that require specific timing of medication dosing to minimize symptoms. Falls and other symptoms such as psychosis and dementia may also occur in more advanced stages of PD, but many of these symptoms can be managed by neurologists or primary care physicians in the outpatient setting. When PD patients are hospitalized, they may not be at a hospital where their neurologist has privileges, or their neurologist may not be consulted. All of these factors impact the care of the hospitalized PD patient. This chapter will discuss the special challenges to managing this population in the inpatient setting.

PD Hospital Admissions and Length of Stay

The reasons for PD hospital admissions can be related to PD motor dysfunction (fluctuations, dyskinesias, imbalance), related to PD non-motor dysfunction (psychiatric symptoms, autonomic dysfunction), indirectly related to PD (i.e., trauma from falls, aspiration pneumonia from dysphagia or side effects from anti-parkinsonian drugs), or non-PD related (i.e., cardiac disorders, genitourinary infection, etc.) (Table 10.1).

PD motor dysfunction is commonly believed to be responsible for the bulk of PD hospital admissions, but most studies list reasons either indirectly related to PD or not related to PD as common reasons for admission, with falls (leading to fractures), cardiac issues/syncope, and infections being the most common.[1–4] Other common reasons for admission include aspiration pneumonia related to dysphagia, encephalopathy/psychiatric issues, nausea/vomiting, neoplasia, stroke, and elective surgeries. One study demonstrated that PD motor

Table 10.1 Reasons for Hospitalization of the PD patient

Category	Examples
PD motor dysfunction	• Motor fluctuations (e.g., wearing-off) • Dyskinesias • Postural instability • Falls
PD non-motor dysfunction	• Cognitive/behavioral disturbances (delirium) • Psychosis • Autonomic dysfunction (OH)
Indirectly related to PD	• Trauma from falls • Aspiration pneumonia from dysphagia • Side effects of antiparkinsonian drugs (nausea/vomiting)
Non-PD related	• Cardiac issues (heart attack, atrial fibrillation) • Stroke/TIA • Urinary tract and other infections • Neoplasm • Elective surgery (e.g., knee replacement)

complications were the primary reason for hospitalization in only 15 percent of the PD patients admitted.[2]

PD patients are hospitalized more frequently than age-matched controls.[5] When admitted, PD patients tend to stay longer (range 2–14 days) than their non-PD counterparts.[6] A substantial number of PD patients have motor deterioration during their hospital stay[7] and when discharged, often require either a short stay at a subacute rehabilitation facility or further outpatient therapy.

Hospitalization-Related Issues and Complications

Medication Management

As PD progresses, patients may develop wearing off (recurrence of parkinsonian symptoms when plasma levodopa levels decrease, typically occurring just before the next dose of medication) and dyskinesias (involuntary choreiform movements affecting any part of the body). In the outpatient setting, neurologists and their PD patients work closely to fine-tune the timing and dosing of medication so that wearing off and dyskinesias are minimized. This results in smooth motor function throughout the day to allow patients to move and perform activities of daily living with few or no limitations. This schedule is often disrupted when PD patients are hospitalized (Table 10.2).

Non-adherence to medication schedules in the inpatient setting is a common problem.[8] This may be purposeful, as patients often need to be N.P.O. for inpatient procedures. However, there may be delays in administering medications for other reasons. This may range from delays in writing admission and medication orders to delays from the pharmacy when sending medications. Medications in the hospital are often ordered using default times. This may be convenient for nursing staff in order to minimize interruptions, but it is often

Table 10.2 Hospitalization-Related Issues and Management Considerations for the Parkinson's Patient

Hospitalization Issues	Management Considerations
Medication Management	• Attempt to adhere to the patient's medication times (write specific times in the orders, rather than number of times per day) or allow the patient to self-administer PD medications. • Ensure the correct formulation of dopaminergic medication (immediate release vs. sustained release) • For PD medications not on the hospital formulary, consider administering the patient's own medication rather than substituting. • Avoid dopamine-blocking agents such as typical and most atypical antipsychotics, and antiemetics such as metoclopramide or prochlorperazine.
Delirium	• Rule out infections or metabolic disturbances and treat appropriately. • Discontinue all centrally active medications if possible. • Implement non-pharmacological treatment measures such as establishing day and night routines and using family and staff to reorient the patient. • If medication is needed, may consider quetiapine or clozapine.
Psychosis	• May be a manifestation of delirium and/or the underlying PD. • PD medications may also cause psychosis. Try discontinuing in the following order: anticholinergic agents, amantadine, MAO-B inhibitors, dopamine agonists, catechol-O-methyltransferase inhibitors, and lastly, levodopa. • If motor symptoms prevent weaning of PD medications, consider quetiapine or clozapine for treatment of psychosis.
Infections	• Aspiration pneumonia (from dysphagia) and urinary tract infections are the most common. • Minimize aspiration risk. • Discontinue Foley catheters. • Treat infections with appropriate antibiotics.
Falls	• Treat orthostatic hypotension if contributing to falls. • Make sure PD medications are given on time. • Consult physical therapy and use assistive devices for those at risk.
Orthostatic Hypotension	• Initiate cardiac evaluation. • Fluid repletion if dehydrated. • Reduce or discontinue anti-hypertensives and dopamine agonists. • If hypotension persists, treat conservatively with salt tabs, thigh-high stockings, and then consider fludrocortisone or midodrine.
Deep Brain Stimulation	• MR: Only brain imaging (i.e., not MR of other locations) can be performed and only using specific guidelines. • DBS may interfere with EKG or EEG and can be turned off during those procedures. • Only bipolar electrocautery should be used during surgery.

not ideal for a patient with PD because of their highly individualized administration schedule. A potential solution is to ensure that the patient's medications are written with specific times ("Take carbidopa/levodopa by mouth at 9 am/12 pm/3 pm/6 pm/9 pm") rather than the number of times a day. Furthermore, many hospitals may have a policy that allows nursing staff to have flexibility in administering medications (generally, one hour before or after a scheduled dose). This makes it easier for the nurse to complete required duties and provides flexibility in case of emergency on the ward, but increases the chance that a PD patient will have erratic timing of medications. This issue should be addressed by educating patients to speak up and educating hospital providers and nursing staff about the importance of maintaining a PD patient's home medication schedule. Competent patients should also be allowed to self-medicate their PD medications if hospital policy will allow.

Inappropriate prescribing may also occur. This may happen because the patient's home medication is unavailable from the hospital pharmacy. As a result, PD medications may be omitted from a patient's regimen, or inappropriate substitutions may occur. A common example is the substitution of the dopamine agonist ropinirole for pramipexole, or vice versa. Another example is the substitution of rotigotine (available in patch form) or apomorphine (an injectable dopamine agonist) for an oral dopamine agonist (ropinirole or pramipexole) when a patient cannot take medications by mouth. Unfortunately, these medications are not easily converted from one dose to another. Additionally, the prescribing inpatient physician may not realize that there are different formulations for levodopa. Immediate-acting carbidopa/levodopa has a different half-life and bioavailability than sustained release carbidopa/levodopa, and substituting one for the other may worsen dyskinesias and wearing off. Clinicians should pay special attention when placing medication orders to ensure the proper formulation is prescribed. When medications are not available from the hospital pharmacy, patients should be allowed to bring in their medications from home to be administered in the hospital.

If the patient cannot take medications by mouth, clinicians should consider placing nasogastric tubes for medication administration. It is important to remember that if dopaminergic medications are abruptly stopped, patients are placed at increased risk of neuroleptic malignant syndrome, characterized by rigidity, high fever, delirium, autonomic instability, and the potential for muscle damage and kidney failure from rhabdomyolysis.

Other medication errors involve the administration of contraindicated medications in those with PD (Table 10.3).

In a survey of PD specialists regarding their perception of hospital care for PD patients, over 70 percent were not confident that hospital staff knew the common medications that worsen PD symptoms.[9] These often include antipsychotic medications (haloperidol, thorazine, risperidone, olanzapine) as well as anti-nausea medications (metoclopramide, prochlorperazine, and promethazine). For nausea, a good alternative is ondansetron, which has no anti-dopaminergic properties. Benzodiazepines may also be used, but they place the patient at increased risk for confusion, delirium, poor balance, and falls. When treating psychosis in a patient with PD, quetiapine or clozapine is

Table 10.3 Medications to Avoid or Limit in PD Patients in the Inpatient Setting (Non-Exhaustive List)

Medications to Avoid:	
Antipsychotics	• Haloperidol
	• Thorazine
	• Risperidone
	• Olanzapine
Select Anti-Nausea Medications/ Anti-Emetics	• Metoclopramide
	• Prochlorperazine
	• Promethazine

Medications to Limit and/or Use with Caution(Particularly if Pre-Existing Cognitive Impairment):	
Narcotics	• Morphine
	• Codeine
	• Oxycodone
Anxiolytics	• Lorazepam
	• Diazepam
Other Hypnotics	• Diphenhydramine
	• Zolpidem
	• Zopiclone
	• Trazodone
	• Amitriptyline
H2-Receptor Blockers	• Ranitidine
	• Cimetidine
	• Famotidine
Muscle Relaxants	• Baclofen
	• Tizanidine
Anticholinergics	• Oxybutynin
	• Tolterodine
	• Trihexyphenidyl
	• Benztropine

preferred (see section on psychosis). Medication management considerations are summarized in Table 10.2.

Delirium

Delirium is a transient, usually reversible, cause of cerebral dysfunction that manifests clinically with a wide range of neuropsychiatric abnormalities, including decreased attention span, and waxing and waning confusion. Unfamiliar places, infection, effects from anesthesia, and changes in medications all can trigger delirium in the hospitalized PD patient. Delirium occurs more often in the elderly and those with preexisting dementia. Understanding and preventing delirium in the hospitalized patient is important, as recent studies have shown that those with delirium have an increased risk of death compared with controls after an average follow-up of 22.7 months (38 percent versus 27.5 percent).[10]

One of the most common causes of delirium in hospitalized PD patients is infection. Typical infections include urinary tract infections, pneumonia, surgical site infections, blood stream infections, and skin infections. PD patients in particular may be at higher risk of pneumonia due to dysphagia.[1–4,6,9]

Another common cause of delirium is medication effect, particularly with medications affecting the central nervous system, such as narcotics, anxiolytics, hypnotics, some antidepressants, antiemetics, H2-receptor blockers, muscle relaxants, and anticholinergics (Table 10.3). When a medication effect is suspected, clinicians should discontinue possible offending agents and simplify the patient's medication regimen as much as possible. In patients with PD, certain anti-parkinsonian drugs may contribute to delirium and should be gradually discontinued or reduced to the lowest possible dose. In patients with PD and dementia, cholinesterase inhibitors such as donepezil should not be abruptly discontinued, as this can exacerbate delirium.

While pain medications, especially narcotics, often contribute to delirium, uncontrolled pain may also contribute. Because of this, the treating team should consistently assess the patient's pain rating and take special care to maintain the fine balance between adequately treating and over-treating pain. One option would be to use non-narcotic pain medication as first line or using the synergistic effect of non-narcotic medications when coupled with small doses of narcotic medication.

For treating delirium, non-pharmacological measures should be tried first. Blinds or drapes should be opened in the daytime, and attempts should be made to keep the patient awake during the day and asleep during the night. Family members should be encouraged to stay and provide familiar cues to help reorient the patient. If patients require further intervention, or if hyperagitated delirium places the patient at increased risk of self-harm, pharmacological treatments could then be considered. Atypical antipsychotics such as clozapine and quetiapine may be an option, though the evidence for these agents in the treatment of delirium is limited.[1,11] These agents are useful if psychosis is part of the delirium (see the section on psychosis). Approaches to managing delirium are summarized in Table 10.2.

Psychosis

Psychosis may occur in up to 40 percent of patients with PD.[12] The psychosis in PD often manifests as visual hallucinations and (less likely) delusions. In the hospital setting, the risk for psychosis is increased by coexisting delirium and disturbances in the sleep–wake cycle. In addition, all of the medications used to treat PD may result in psychosis. If the patient's development of psychosis seems to fit temporally with the increase or addition of dopaminergic medications, these medications should be decreased or gradually discontinued. Typically, levodopa preparations cause less psychosis than the other anti-parkinsonian agents, so anti-parkinsonian medications should be discontinued in the following order: anticholinergic agents (e.g. trihexyphenidyl), amantadine, MAO-B inhibitors, dopamine agonists, catechol-O-methyltransferase (COMT) inhibitors and, finally, levodopa[12] (Table 10.2).

Although discontinuing or reducing PD medications may ameliorate psychotic symptoms in some cases, patients may not be able to tolerate these changes because of worsening motor function. If psychosis persists despite decreasing anti-parkinsonian medications to the lowest possible level, additional pharmacotherapy may be necessary. Cholinesterase inhibitors such as donepezil or rivastigmine may be helpful for psychosis in some patients and are usually well tolerated, though worsened tremor is a potential side effect. If an antipsychotic is necessary, only quetiapine or clozapine should be considered. All other atypical antipsychotics as well as typical antipsychotics (e.g., haloperidol) should be avoided because they worsen motor function. Clozapine is an atypical antipsychotic that, at doses of 6.25 to 50 mg/d, reduces psychotic symptoms without worsening motor symptoms.[13] However, there is a risk of developing agranulocytosis with clozapine, which often leads to prescriber hesitancy in using this medication. When used, routine monitoring of the complete blood count is needed. Quetiapine is more often prescribed first for psychosis in PD, but the data for quetiapine in treating psychosis in PD is not as good as for clozapine.[14]

Elective Surgery and Anesthesia

Just like any other patient, PD patients may require hospitalization for elective surgery. Considerations when planning inpatient or outpatient surgery are summarized in Table 10.4.

Elective general and orthopedic procedures in those with PD are associated with longer hospital stays, higher in-hospital mortality, and increased post-operative complications such as bacterial infections when compared to those without PD.[15] There is also increased risk of post-operative falls, especially among trauma-related admissions. Medical optimization by a neurologist, early mobilization, physical therapy, and careful monitoring for post-operative complications may help optimize surgical outcomes.[16]

It is common for patients to experience post-operative nausea with elective surgery. Anti-emetics such as metoclopramide or prochlorperazine are often ordered as part of a default post-operative order set. Unfortunately, these medications have similar chemical structures to the antipsychotics and should be avoided in those with PD. Domperidone (not available in the United States), trimethobenzamide, ondansetron, dolasetron, and granisetron are acceptable substitutes for nausea in the PD patient.

Post-operative delirium is also common after elective surgery. Delirium in this setting should be treated like any delirium (see the section on delirium). Patients and their family should be warned that delirium is possible after surgical procedures. With anticipatory guidance, delirium may be more easily managed.

If possible, PD medications should be continued up to the time of surgery and restarted immediately in the post-operative period in order to minimize worsening of motor function. Care must be taken to avoid post-operative ileus,

Table 10.4 Considerations When Planning Elective Surgery in the Parkinson's Disease Patient

Issue	Management Considerations
Preoperative Counseling	• Patients and families should discuss PD medication management with surgeon. • PD patients may have longer recovery times from certain surgeries, particularly those affecting mobilization. • Increased risk of delirium in hospitalized PD patients post-operatively, particularly in patients with pre-existing cognitive impairment.
Home Medication Management	• Continue all PD medications, including on day of surgery. • Minimize missed doses of PD medications; restart home medications immediately post-operatively. • If patients cannot take oral medications post-operatively, place nasogastric tube early to minimize missed doses. • Never stop PD medications abruptly, given risk of neuroleptic malignant syndrome.
Anesthesia	• Avoid general anesthesia if possible. • Avoid thiopental sodium.
Management of Other Perioperative Medications	• Review routine/standard operative medication sets to make sure there are no medications that should be avoided in PD patients (e.g., certain antiemetics, diphenhydramine). • Do not use antiemetics such as metoclopramide or prochlorperazine for nausea, given risk of worsening parkinsonism. • Balance pain control and risk of delirium by using minimum needed narcotics and combining these medications with non-narcotic pain management options. • Avoid other medications that may contribute to delirium or worsen cognitive function (see Table 10.2).
Postoperative Management	• Aggressive prevention and management of postoperative ileus. • Early mobilization and physical therapy. • Early planning for rehabilitation.
Other	• Low threshold for consulting neurology.

as Parkinson's medications are generally not available parenterally. While dopamine agonist patches (rotigotine) and apomorphine (which is given by injection) are available if a patient cannot take medications orally, there is no commonly accepted conversion formula to safely switch patients to these formulations. If possible, nasogastric tubes should be inserted as soon as possible in order to administer PD medications, as sudden discontinuation of PD medications increases the risk of neuroleptic malignant syndrome.

We prefer that a PD patient receive regional anesthesia for their elective surgery, if possible. While there are limited data on the type of surgical anesthesia that is optimal for PD, the use of regional anesthesia avoids the after-effects of general anesthesia, such as nausea, sedation, and confusion.[17] General anesthesia may also put a PD patient at higher risk of pneumonia if the patient has dysphagia or difficulty clearing secretions. There are no clear recommendations on which general anesthetic drugs should be used in PD. However, thiopental sodium should probably be avoided as an induction agent because of case reports that it can worsen parkinsonism.[18]

Infections

Infections, especially aspiration pneumonia, are a common reason for hospitalization in PD.[1–4,6,9] PD patients are at increased risk of aspiration due to dysphagia and poor control of secretions secondary to motor dysfunction. Careful measures to reduce aspiration risk include making sure PD patients get proper medication doses on time and obtaining input from a speech-language pathologist, who may suggest altering meal consistency, employing chin-tucking maneuvers or inserting a feeding tube. It is important to note that feeding tubes do not decrease the risk of aspiration but make it easier to administer medications. Swallowing ability should be assessed soon after taking dopaminergic medications, when the patient is in an optimal motor state. Once patients with PD are suspected to have pneumonia, appropriate care must be provided promptly to help decrease delirium risk. The organisms responsible for pneumonia in PD are similar to those responsible for the illness in the general population.

Urinary tract infections are also common in the PD population. Not every patient will be symptomatic and develop urgency, dysuria, or frequency, so clinicians should have a low threshold for ordering a urinalysis, especially if delirium is present. General preventative measures include early removal of Foley catheters and intermittent straight catheterization if necessary. Preventative measures are also critical to prevent skin infections, as patients with PD often have prolonged hospitalizations and coexisting motor dysfunction. Care must be taken by the clinicians and support staff to ensure proper turning techniques and general measures to help prevent skin breakdown and bedsores.

PD patients commonly observe that their parkinsonian motor symptoms worsen with infections. When the infection is treated and resolves, their motor symptoms return to baseline. Thus, all infections in PD patients should be treated aggressively. There is no clear evidence that antibiotics worsen PD.

Falls and Trauma

One of the leading causes for hospital admission in PD patients appears to be falls and trauma, suggesting that fall prevention may prevent hospital admissions.[2,5,6] Unfortunately, falls are common in PD, and the majority occur during walking, stopping, turning, standing up, or bending down[19]. They rarely occur secondary to slipping or tripping. PD patients often report difficulty stopping or turning in small spaces and also may have freezing of gait (a sudden cessation of movement when walking). In later stages of PD, postural instability (or loss of the postural righting reflexes) may occur. All of these problems may predispose the PD patient to falling. Up to 40 percent of patients with postural instability have multiple falls that predispose them to injury, including wrist and hip fractures.[20]

When a PD patient is admitted because of multiple falls, optimization of dopaminergic medications may help, especially if the cause is bradykinesia or motor fluctuations. Unfortunately, postural instability, when it develops, is often refractory to dopaminergic treatment. Avoidance of contraindicated medications and keeping the home medication schedule may prevent deterioration while hospitalized. Physical therapy consultation as an inpatient may also be helpful in teaching the patient strategies to promote postural stability and prevent falls, as well as to assess the need for ambulatory aids such as canes or walkers.

When a PD patient is admitted with a hip fracture, early mobilization is essential to restore previous function in as short a time as possible. Neurological consultation is also recommended to prevent a lengthy stay. Finally, the measures recommended in earlier sections to prevent infection and delirium should be followed (Table 10.2).

Orthostatic Hypotension

Lightheadedness when standing, or orthostatic hypotension (OH), is a common complaint among the aging population. It is often defined as a drop in blood pressure by 20 mmHg from lying to standing at 3 minutes, or an increase in pulse by 10 beats per minute after 3 minutes of standing. Dehydration, vasoactive medications, or diuretics are common etiologies. In PD, OH is a common non-motor feature and results from a loss of post-synaptic noradrenergic neurons, which later leads to impaired sympathetic input to the cardiovascular system.[21]

Before attributing OH to the disease itself, dehydration should be considered and fluid repletion initiated if not contraindicated. A cardiac evaluation should also be performed, including inpatient telemetry monitoring and possibly cardiology consultation with echocardiogram or tilt-table testing. Strong consideration should be given to discontinuing anti-hypertensives. OH can also result from PD medications. Among these, dopamine agonists are the most likely contributor and often have a dose-dependent effect. Gradually discontinuing PD medications, especially dopamine agonists, or reducing them to the lowest tolerated dose, may help OH.

Once orthostasis from dehydration or cardiac cause has been excluded and contributing medications have been reduced or discontinued, additional measures can be considered (Table 10.2). Nonpharmacological treatments include avoiding quick rises from a prone or seated position, squatting, crossing legs, and tensing the abdomen, legs, or buttocks to increase venous flow to the heart, thigh-high compression stockings, and increased salt intake from salt tablets (>8 grams daily). Pharmacological agents include midodrine 2.5–10 mg three times daily and fludrocortisone 0.1–0.3 mg daily.

Particular Considerations in the DBS Patient

As discussed in the prior chapter, deep brain stimulation (DBS) is an effective surgical treatment for appropriate PD patients. While the PD patient with DBS will have many of the same problems as the PD patient without DBS mentioned above, there are a few considerations that apply only to someone with a DBS system.

X-rays, computed tomography, and ultrasound procedures can be performed in someone with a DBS system, but there are limitations with MR imaging. The risk of MR imaging in an individual with DBS includes heating, device disruption, and induced electrical current that might lead to brain tissue damage.[22] In order to minimize the risks of MR imaging, only brain MR imaging can be performed in patients with DBS. According to Medtronic Inc., the only provider of FDA-approved DBS systems in the United States, this should be done using a 1.5–Tesla MR machine with a receive-only head coil or head transmit coil. Other technical specifications include not exceeding a head SAR value of 0.1 W/kg and limiting the gradient switching (dB/dt) to $\leq$ 20 T/sec. Because of these restrictions, some hospitals may not perform MR imaging in patients with a DBS system. With older neurostimulator models (Kinetra, Soletra), the stimulator should be programmed to 0 volts, then turned off before the MRI. If the stimulator settings are maintained and not turned down to 0 volts, the MRI may toggle the stimulator on and off and cause uncomfortable sensations in the patient. Someone familiar with DBS will need to turn the stimulator down to 0 volts as the patient's own handheld device will not turn the voltage down, though the patient device is able to turn the stimulator off and on. With newer models (Activa PC, Activa SC), the patient's own handheld device can turn the voltage down and turn the neurostimulator off.

The DBS system can also interfere with the ability to obtain an electrocardiogram (ECG) or electroencephalogram (EEG), by introducing artifacts into the tracing. However, the stimulator can be simply turned off prior to performing the test and turned on immediately after the test. This can be done with the patient's own handheld device. While the patient may be uncomfortable with the DBS system off, they usually can tolerate it for the length of the test without significant problems.

Some precautions are also necessary for the DBS patient undergoing elective surgery. Electrocautery during surgery may damage the lead or extension. It may also temporarily stop the output of the stimulator and even reset it to its default settings. When electrocautery is necessary during surgery, bipolar electrocautery is recommended, with the ground plate kept as far away from the DBS system as possible. If possible, the stimulator should be checked after surgery to confirm that the stimulator is on and that the settings are correct. Coordinating elective surgeries with the patient's DBS team can help facilitate post-operative checking of the system.

Improving Care of the Hospitalized PD Patient

As outlined in this chapter, there are many unique challenges in managing the PD patient in the hospital. Patients are generally dissatisfied with their in-hospital care, and hospital providers may be unfamiliar with the special considerations needed to help them care for these patients. While there are no studies on which interventions improve the hospital care of patients with PD, many reviews and commentary papers by experts in the field advocate early consultation with a neurologist and getting neurologists to facilitate urgent follow-up appointments after discharge. Improving educational outreach on the timing of PD medications to patients and families, hospital nurses, and non-neurologist physicians in the community has also been recommended. To that end, Parkinson's UK, a patient-advocacy organization in the United Kingdom, initiated a "Get It on Time" campaign with the goal of educating patients and hospital and long-term care staff about the importance of medication timing in PD. Similarly, the National Parkinson Foundation, a major patient advocacy organization in the United States, started the "Aware In Care" program, focused towards patients with PD to help them get the best care possible during a hospital stay. These programs are a good start, but the current practice must also change from a hospital-provider standpoint for long-lasting improvement.

References

1. Klein C, Prokhorov T, Miniovitz A, Dobronevsky E, Rabey JM. Admission of Parkinsonian patients to a neurological ward in a community hospital. *J Neural Transm.* Nov 2009;116(11):1509–1512.

2. Temlett JA, Thompson PD. Reasons for admission to hospital for Parkinson's disease. *Intern Med J.* Aug 2006;36(8):524–526.

3. Vossius C, Nilsen OB, Larsen JP. Parkinson's disease and hospital admissions: frequencies, diagnoses and costs. *Acta Neurol Scand.* Jan 2010;121(1):38–43.

4. Woodford H, Walker R. Emergency hospital admissions in idiopathic Parkinson's disease. *Mov Disord.* Sep 2005;20(9):1104–1108.

5. Guttman M, Slaughter PM, Theriault ME, DeBoer DP, Naylor CD. Burden of parkinsonism: a population-based study. *Mov Disord.* Mar 2003;18(3):313–319.

6. Gerlach OH, Winogrodzka A, Weber WE. Clinical problems in the hospitalized Parkinson's disease patient: systematic review. *Mov Disord.* Feb 1 2011;26(2):197–208.

7. Gerlach OH, Broen MP, van Domburg PH, Vermeij AJ, Weber WE. Deterioration of Parkinson's disease during hospitalization: survey of 684 patients. *BMC Neurol.* 2012;12:13.

8. Magdalinou KN, Martin A, Kessel B. Prescribing medications in Parkinson's disease (PD) patients during acute admissions to a District General Hospital. *Parkinsonism Relat Disord.* Dec 2007;13(8):539–540.

9. Chou KL, Zamudio J, Schmidt P, et al. Hospitalization in Parkinson's disease: a survey of National Parkinson Foundation Centers. *Parkinsonism Relat Disord.* Jul 2011;17(6):440–445.

10. Witlox J, Eurelings LS, de Jonghe JF, Kalisvaart KJ, Eikelenboom P, van Gool WA. Delirium in elderly patients and the risk of postdischarge mortality, institutionalization, and dementia: a meta-analysis. *JAMA.* Jul 28 2010;304(4):443–451.

11. Khouzam HR. Quetiapine in the treatment of postoperative delirium. A report of three cases. *Compr Ther.* Fall–Winter 2008;34(3–4):207–217.

12. Chou KL, Fernandez HH. Combating psychosis in Parkinson's disease patients: the use of antipsychotic drugs. *Expert Opin Invest Drugs.* Apr 2006;15(4):339–349.

13. Wood LD, Neumiller JJ, Setter SM, Dobbins EK. Clinical review of treatment options for select nonmotor symptoms of Parkinson's disease. *Am J Geriatr Pharmacother.* Aug 2010;8(4):294–315.

14. Miyasaki JM, Shannon K, Voon V, et al. Practice parameter: evaluation and treatment of depression, psychosis, and dementia in Parkinson's disease (an evidence-based review): report of the Quality Standards Subcommittee of the American Academy of Neurology. *Neurology.* Apr 11 2006;66(7):996–1002.

15. Aminoff MJ, Christine CW, Friedman JH, et al. Management of the hospitalized patient with Parkinson's disease: current state of the field and need for guidelines. *Parkinsonism Relat Disord.* Mar 2011;17(3):139–145.

16. Mehta S, Vankleunen JP, Booth RE, Lotke PA, Lonner JH. Total knee arthroplasty in patients with Parkinson's disease: impact of early postoperative neurologic intervention. *Am J Orthop (Belle Mead NJ).* Oct 2008;37(10):513–516.

17. Nicholson G, Pereira AC, Hall GM. Parkinson's disease and anaesthesia. *Br J Anaesth.* Dec 2002;89(6):904–916.

18. Muravchick S, Smith DS. Parkinsonian symptoms during emergence from general anesthesia. *Anesthesiology.* Jan 1995;82(1):305–307.

19. Bloem BR, Grimbergen YA, Cramer M, Willemsen M, Zwinderman AH. Prospective assessment of falls in Parkinson's disease. *J Neurol.* Nov 2001;248(11):950–958.

20. Gray P, Hildebrand K. Fall risk factors in Parkinson's disease. *J Neurosci Nurs.* Aug 2000;32(4):222–228.

21. Sharabi Y, Goldstein DS. Mechanisms of orthostatic hypotension and supine hypertension in Parkinson's disease. *J Neurol Sci.* Nov 15 2011;310(1–2):123–128.

22. Rezai AR, Baker KB, Tkach JA, et al. Is magnetic resonance imaging safe for patients with neurostimulation systems used for deep brain stimulation? *Neurosurgery.* Nov 2005;57(5):1056–1062; discussion 1056–1062.

Chapter 11

Management of Late Complications of Parkinson's Disease

Jennifer Singerman and Janis Miyasaki

The World Health Organization defines *palliative care* as "an approach that improves the quality of life (QoL) of patients and their families facing the problem associated with life-threatening illness, through the prevention and relief of suffering by means of early identification and impeccable assessment and treatment of pain and other problems, physical, psychosocial and spiritual."[1] Although it is a common misperception that palliative care should be equated with end-of-life treatment, the main goal is to provide comfort and treatment of symptoms that affect QoL, regardless of illness stage. Parkinson's disease requires much symptom management, particularly as the disease progresses and disability increases.

The mean annual rate of progression of motor disability in PD patients is 2.7–7.4 percent when using the Unified Parkinson's Disease Rating Scale (UPDRS) motor section and Hoehn and Yahr stage.[2] Motor progression slows with longer follow-up. Complications such as dyskinesias, motor fluctuations, falls, and neuropsychiatric symptoms worsen with advancing disease.

In addition to morbidity, PD confers an additional mortality risk. In the pre-levodopa era, the mortality of PD patients was three times that of expected.[3] A more recent study showed that treated PD patients have a mortality rate of 1.52 above age-matched controls.[4] Aspiration pneumonia is the most common cause of death in PD, with nearly half of patients succumbing to this complication.[5]

Optimum palliative care delivery uses an interdisciplinary team. In addition to a neurologist, a palliative care physician, nurse specialist, care coordinator and spiritual counselor should be available to patients and families. The team approach ensures that patients and families receive a comprehensive assessment, consistent information and advice, and a holistic care plan. Toronto Western Hospital Movement Disorders Centre has had such a team for the past five years. In the following chapter, we will share helpful practice points based on the inaugural period at this clinic.

In the absence of a comprehensive team, many palliative care concepts can be translated to either a neurological practice or primary-care practice setting. Attention to non-motor PD symptoms, inclusion of the family in the care plan, and education regarding the expected disease trajectory can relieve patient and family suffering and reframe disability and progression. While non-motor symptoms are also discussed in Chapter 7, some are re-discussed here to guide clinicians on aspects critical to managing patients with late complications of PD.

Specific Issues in Patients with Advanced Parkinson's Disease

Top concerns in advanced PD patients include fluctuating medication response, mood, drooling, and sleep (Table 11.1). Pain was the sixth most common complaint in these patients.[6] Bowel and bladder problems, which may not be discussed due to clinician or patient discomfort, were common and have a large impact on QoL.

Constipation

Constipation can precede motor manifestations of PD by many years. Additionally, poor mobility is independently associated with constipation. PD severity is associated with incomplete emptying at defecation, need for assisted defecation, and unsuccessful defecation attempts.[7] Constipation severity is associated with advanced

Table 11.1 Most common symptoms in advanced PD[6]	
Rank	Symptom
1	Motor fluctuations
2	Mood
3	Drooling
4	Sleep
5	Tremor
6	Pain
7	Bowel complaints
8	Urinary dysfunction
9	Falls
10	Appetite/weight loss
11	Slowness
12	Fatigue
13	Sexual dysfunction
14	Hallucinations/delusions
-	Restless legs
-	Speech
17	Compulsive behavior
18	Handwriting
-	Loss of smell/taste
-	Sweating
21	Stiffness
-	Swallowing
23	Freezing
-	Memory

Hoehn and Yahr stage and time since diagnosis, but not with age, gender, or age at diagnosis. The number of unsuccessful defecation attempts is higher in patients not currently on levodopa treatment, possibly related to external anal sphincter dystonia. Because constipation is so common and impacts QoL, an aggressive bowel routine including stool softeners and laxatives should be employed (Table 11.2). Dietary changes such as natural sources of fiber, increased vegetable and fruit intake, and reduced intake of refined carbohydrates can be helpful. Polyethylene glycol 3350 (PEG 3350), a laxative usually used to clean out the bowel in preparation for colonoscopy, can be used in the setting of severe, chronic constipation in PD to increase bowel movements and reduce associated pain.[8]

Pain

In a study of 176 PD patients, 83 percent experienced pain, identified as four major types: (1) musculoskeletal pain as a result of rigidity or skeletal deformities; (2) dystonic pain, often secondary to levodopa-induced dyskinesias; (3) radicular-neuropathic pain; and (4) central neuropathic pain.[9] While most patients experienced just one pain type, a significant proportion experienced multiple types.

Pain is often experienced as an "off" phenomenon responding to levodopa treatment. Dystonia is a common cause of "off"-time pain. While levodopa can relieve this symptom early in PD, injections of botulinum toxin may be needed in later PD stages and can also be used to prevent contractures. Neuropathic pain medications can be tried for central or peripheral neuropathic pain (Table 11.2). Musculoskeletal pain is usually the result of immobility and rigidity. Improving "on" time is helpful, but physiotherapy and gentle exercises

Table 11.2 Medications and Typical Dose Ranges for Pharmacological Management	
Constipation	Docusate sodium: 100–300 mg bid
	Senna: 1–4 tabs qhs
	Lactulose: 15–30 mg daily-bid
	PEG: 3350–17 g (~1 heaping tablespoon) mixed into 4–8 oz of fluid daily, can be titrated to daily bowel movements
Pain	Gabapentin: 300–1200 mg tid
	Pregabalin: 75–300 mg bid
	Morphine: 5–10 mg q4h prn, may increase slowly as needed (no ceiling dose but be cautious of cognitive side effects and constipation)
	Botulinum toxin A: Doses vary, for example 20–60 U injected into foot to treat "striatal toe," extension of great toe
Dementia	Rivastigmine: 1.5–6mg bid (or transdermal patch)
	Donepezil: 5–10mg daily
	Galantamine: 4–12mg bid
Psychosis	Quetiapine: 12.5–400mg, typically at night, may add smaller morning dose
	Clozapine: 6.25–50mg/d

for range of motion are important. Family members and caregivers can help with this task.

Although non-pharmacological pain management is preferable, patients often require analgesics. A step-wise approach should be undertaken, with non-opioid analgesics such as acetaminophen or ibuprofen used first. If pain is insufficiently controlled, opioids can be added under physician supervision.

Psychosis and Delirium

Neuropsychiatric symptoms are common non-motor findings in PD. Cognitive impairment in PD tends to have prominent executive dysfunction and visuo-spatial deficits rather than frank memory loss or language difficulty. Visual hallucinations are common. These tend to be well-formed and often consist of animals, small children, or long-deceased relatives who are silent. Many times they are not bothersome to the patient, though they can become distressing. Complicating the picture further, dopaminergic medications can precipitate or worsen neuropsychiatric symptoms.

A multi-tiered approach should be used when treating these symptoms. If there is a new cognitive or behavioral change, an underlying cause should be sought. Infections or metabolic derangements are common causes of delirium. Some anti-parkinsonian medications, such as amantadine and anticholinergic medications, can cause or worsen cognitive impairment and should be discontinued if it occurs. If motor symptoms allow, dopaminergic medications can be reduced somewhat. Non-PD medications can also contribute to cognitive impairment (Table 7.3) and should be discontinued if present. If no reversible cause are elicited, several medications can be tried. Cholinesterase inhibitors are often useful (Table 11.2),[10] and can treat the psychiatric symptoms in addition to cognitive impairment.[11] If psychotic symptoms persist despite cholinesterase inhibitor treatment, antipsychotics (neuroleptics) can be tried. Most of these medications can worsen PD motor symptoms (or even cause paradoxical agitation or neuroleptic malignant syndrome), including "atypical" neuroleptics such as risperidone and olanzepine. The only neuroleptics that should be used in patients with PD are quetiapine or clozapine (Table 11.2).[12] Clozapine carries the risk of agranulocytosis and regular blood monitoring is required.

Withdrawal of Dopaminergic Therapy

Patients often end up on a "cocktail" of several anti-parkinsonian medications accumulating after years of treatment. Some medications started early become less useful or even have harmful side effects as patients progress. Anticholinergics have only a weak anti-parkinsonian effects and can cause significant cognitive impairment; they should be discontinued for any cognitive concerns. Similarly, amantadine can have cognitive side effects. Dopamine agonists and MAO-B inhibitors are useful but are not as effective as levodopa, and they are often discontinued at this stage in favor of increasing levodopa doses.

Levodopa is the mainstay of treatment for PD, but its downsides include motor fluctuations, dyskinesias, and worsening of autonomic symptoms (e.g. orthostatic hypotension) and neuropsychiatric symptoms (e.g. cognitive impairment, delusions, and hallucinations). Many clinicians choose to withdraw dopaminergic medications, including levodopa, once patients reach advanced stages of the disease, particularly if bedridden. A small randomized controlled trial of minimally mobile dementing nursing home residents with PD comparing continuation versus withdrawal of levodopa[10] found that there were no changes in motor function in either group. Cognition and behavior did not worsen in either group, but two of the six patients in the weaning group showed improvements in cognition. This is in contrast to other evidence showing worsening motor function and poorer performance on delayed response tasks with withdrawal of dopaminergic treatment.[13]

Parkinsonian symptoms affect caregivers as well. Severe rigidity makes hygiene difficult. Therefore, there may be advantages to continuing treatment even in patients with minimal mobility. If oral medications are tolerated and delirium is not present, oral dopaminergic medications should generally be continued. If use of oral formulations is impossible but dopaminergic withdrawal results in painful dystonia, rectal levodopa can be considered.[14] To prepare this, grind 100 mg of levodopa into a fine powder and mix with 5 mL of water and 5 mL of glycerol. The mixture needs to be acidified using 1g of citric acid, and can then be infused rectally using the patient's regular dose (1 mL = 100/25 mg of levodopa/carbidopa). Extra solution may be refrigerated in an amber container (to prevent solution breakdown) and shaken well before redosing. If delirium is present, we recommend discontinuing levodopa and treating with quetiapine.

Poor Nutritional Status

Advanced PD patients tend to lose weight, and poor nutritional status contributes to medical complications such as pressure ulcers and infections. Moreover, the most common cause of death in PD is pneumonia, usually related to aspiration. While some patients can be maintained on a modified diet, the question of percutaneous endoscopic gastrostomy (PEG) tube feeding is often raised. Neurological conditions are the most common reason for PEG insertion.[15] Advocates of PEG feeding state that it results in weight gain, reduced incidence of pneumonia, and improvement in QoL.[16] However, PEG feeding does not prolong life or promote wound healing.[17] Tube feeding does not eliminate aspiration risk, as patients still aspirate oral secretions. A feeding tube should not be placed for aspiration alone.[18] Any discussion about feeding tube placement should include indications for stopping enteral feeding. We suggest that the main indication for feeding tube placement should be prolonged feeding time due to dysphagia associated with weight loss and reduced QoL.

Other solutions to poor nutritional status in demented patients have been considered.[17] High-calorie diet supplements improved weight gain but not cognition, mortality, or overall functioning. Appetite stimulants, assisted feeding, and enhanced dietician care resulted in weight gain but did not improve other measures.

Caregiver Burnout

At some point, most PD patients require help with activities of daily living. These caregiving demands typically fall on family, often a spouse. Caregiver burden increases proportionally with the amount of care a patient requires.

In addition to total amount of care, psychiatric symptoms are associated with increasing caregiver demand.[19] Because PD is a slowly progressive disease, it can be difficult to determine when further services are needed, and therefore they are often not offered. This increases stress and furthers caregiver burnout.

When caregivers of PD patients were interviewed regarding caring for advanced PD patients,[20] the main themes were caregivers' role and burden, palliative care, bereavement, and access to health and social care services. Many caregivers felt that they were forced to take on several roles, including nurse, pharmacist, and secretary, without any helpful direction from medical professionals. Their own QoL was compromised and they were unable to make plans or do things for themselves. This often resulted in a crisis situation where the patient was placed urgently in an inpatient facility to provide respite for the caregiver. When patients ultimately passed away, many caregivers felt unprepared to deal with the death and had in the meantime become quite socially isolated, making it harder to cope. This highlights the importance of providing caregivers with adequate information about the disease and its progression and access to services to make their role easier.

Hospice Referral

PD patients are less likely to die at home than other elderly patients (9 percent vs. 17 percent)[21] with a trend towards end-of-life hospital admission; 63 percent of PD patients dying in hospital were admitted from home. No patients in this study[21] died in hospice, but 36 percent died in a care home (versus 21 percent of the control population). If more palliative services had been offered to these patients, some of the hospital admissions might have been avoided. In our center, which provides ambulatory palliative care services, of 145 patients followed, 27 have died and only three died in an acute care hospital setting.

Conclusions

Many motor, cognitive, psychiatric, and emotional issues affect advanced PD patients and their caregivers. End-stage PD issues are manageable if they are given the attention that they deserve.

References

1. WHO Definition of Palliative Care. World Health Organization website. Available at http://www.who.int/cancer/palliative/definition/en/, updated 2012. Accessed August 30, 2012.

2. Schrag A, Dodel R, Spottke A, Bornschein B, Siebert U, Quinn NP. Rate of clinical progression in Parkinson's disease. A prospective study. *Mov Disord*. 2007;22(7):938–945.

3. Hoehn MM, Yahr MD. Parkinsonism: onset, progression and mortality. *Neurology*. 1967;17(5):427.

4. Herlofson K, Lie SA, Arsland D, Larsen JP. Mortality and Parkinson's disease: a community-based study. *Neurology*. 2004;62:937–942.

5. Pennington S, Snell K, Lee M, Walker R. The cause of death in idiopathic Parkinson's disease. *Parkinsonism Relat Disord.* 2010;16(7):434–437.

6. Politis M, Wu K, Molloy S, Bain PG, Chaudhuri KR, Piccini P. Parkinson's disease symptoms: the patient's perspective. *Mov Disord.* 2010;25(11):1646–1651.

7. Krogh K, Ostergaard K, Sabroe S, Laurberg S. Clinical aspects of bowel symptoms in Parkinson's disease. *Acta Neurol Scand.* 2008;117(1):60–64.

8. Gruss JH, Ulm G. Efficacy and tolerability of PEG 3350 plus electrolytes (Movicol®) in chronic constipation associated with Parkinson's disease. *Euro J Ger.* 2004;6(3):143–150.

9. Beiske AG, Loge JH, Rønningen A, Svensson E. Pain in Parkinson's disease: prevalence and characteristics. Pain. 2009;141(1–2):173–177.

10. Emre M, Aarsland D, Albanese A, et al. Rivastigmine for dementia associated with Parkinson's disease. *N Engl J Med.* 2004;351(24):2509.

11. Aarsland D, Hutchinson M, Larsen JP. Cognitive, psychiatric and motor response to galantamine in Parkinson's disease with dementia. *Int J Geriatr Psychiatry.* 2003;18(10):937.

12. Miyasaki JM, Shannon K, Voon V, et al. Practice parameter: evaluation and treatment of depression, psychosis, and dementia in Parkinson's disease (an evidence-based review): Report of the Quality Standards Subcommittee of the American Academy of Neurology. Neurology. 2006;66;996.

13. Fern-Pollak L, Whone AL, Brooks DJ, et al. Cognitive and motor effects of do-paminergic medication withdrawal in Parkinson's disease. *Neuropsychologia.* 2004;24:1917–1926.

14. Cooper SD, Ismail HA, Frank C. Case report: successful use of rectally administered levodopa-carbidopa. *Can Fam Physician.* 2001;47:112–113.

15. Kurien M, Westaby D, Romaya C, Sanders DS. National survey evaluating service provision for percutaneous endoscopic gastrostomy within the UK. *Scand J Gastroenterol.* 2011;46(12):1519–1524.

16. Britton JE, Lipscomb G, Mohr PD, Rees WD, Young AC. The use of percutaneous endoscopic gastrostomy (PEG) feeding tubes in patients with neurological disease. *J Neurol.* 1997;244(7):431–434.

17. Hanson LC, Ersek M, Gilliam R, Carey TS. Oral feeding options for people with dementia: a systematic review. *J Am Geriatr Soc.* 2011;59(3):463–4672.

18. Finucane TE, Christmas C, Travis K. Tube feeding in patients with advanced dementia: a review of the evidence. *JAMA.* 1999;282(14):1365–1370.

19. Schrag A, Hovris A, Morley D, Quinn N, Jahanshahi M. Caregiver-burden in Parkinson's disease is closely associated with psychiatric symptoms, falls and disability. *Parkinsonism Relat Disord.* 2003;12:35–41.

20. Hasson F, Kernohan WG, McLaughlin M, et al. An exploration into the palliative and end-of-life experiences of carers of people with Parkinson's disease. *Palliat Med.* 2010;24(7):731–736.

21. Snell K, Pennington S, Lee M, Walker R. The place of death in Parkinson's disease. *Age Ageing.* 38(5);2009:617–619.

Chapter 12

The Role of the Non-Physician: Rehabilitation and Non-Pharmacological Therapy in Parkinson's Disease

Jason S. Hawley

Many patients with Parkinson's disease are interested in exploring all avenues of treatment. Physicians frequently discuss patient's questions about exercise, therapy, vitamins, and nutrition. These therapies are often referred to as "non-pharmacological" therapies, and they are increasingly playing a role in the symptomatic treatment of PD. In many locations, there are therapists who focus on treating Parkinson's disease, and provide competent and specialized therapy to their patients. Moreover, there is increasing evidence for the effectiveness of these non-pharmacological therapies both for treating the symptoms of PD as well as improving the quality of life for patients with PD. This chapter will focus on three therapies—physical therapy, occupational therapy, and speech therapy. We will discuss these treatment modalities, which can be safe, effective, and in some cases add significantly to improving function, reducing disability, and improving the psychological burden of the PD.

Exercise and Physical Therapy in PD

The distinction between "exercise" and "physical therapy" frequently relates to the degree of functional disability. Individuals with early PD who are still working and very active will ask about exercise, and may not believe they require a physical therapist. On the other hand, more disabled individuals with long-standing PD may require physical therapy, with "exercise" being too dangerous, given their functional limitations. These distinctions are mainly semantic, because it is clear that focused physiotherapy can be beneficial in early, middle, and late stages of PD, and physical therapists are important contributors to the care of many individuals with PD. Moreover, with different types of physical therapy treatments available, a focused understanding at a basic level is necessary, as many of our patients participate in these activities, often at their own initiative. We will address three different types—physiotherapy, movement strategy training with cuing devices, and formalized patterned exercises. These modalities are described in Table 12.1.[1]

Most evidence for the role of exercise and physical therapy is in studies examining standard physiotherapy. While there is significant variability in techniques of therapy, study population, and outcome measures, the overall evidence suggests that standard physiotherapy can improve balance and motor functioning in patients with PD. As balance and gait impairments are among the most predictive measures of disability in PD, modalities that preserve gait function are very important to the long-term management of PD.[2] It is recommended that therapists use exercises that focus on maintaining balance and gait training in mild to moderate PD. Sustained walking, treadmill training, or using machines that focus on the repetitive action of the legs can be useful. Balance exercises that target moving the center of mass, narrowing the gait, and providing challenging balance exercises are most beneficial. It is notable that while physiotherapy has improved balance and gait metrics (for example, stride length and stride variability), it has not been shown to prevent falls. This is an important distinction for clinicians to keep in mind when referring patients for physiotherapy. Moreover, it further suggests that the physiology of gait control (speed, stride length, stability), may be slightly different from the physiology of postural control and the mechanism related to falling in PD. The role of physiotherapy should therefore be targeted at improved gait function, and may not be beneficial for the individual with PD who has frequent falls.[1]

Three recent studies have examined the role of cueing or using focused attention to assist patients with PD affected by gait freezing and falling. The study population in these samples had more advanced PD. While training methods using cueing did mildly improve UPDRS scores and specific gait metrics, the overall clinical impact appeared small. As with any physical therapy modalities, one of the most important issues is sustainability of the intervention. In a three-month follow-up after the intervention, it was clear that the improvements were not sustained.[3,4] The usefulness of cueing and therapies that used

Table 12.1 Modalities of Physical Therapy Used and Studied in PD		
Modality:	**Description**	**Examples**
Physiotherapy	Stretching, walking, or using conventional exercise equipment under the guidance of a specialized physical therapist.	−Treadmill training −Home-based exercise programs −Supervised physical therapy at varying degrees of intensity
Movement Strategy Training with Cueing Devices	Cueing is a technique whereby external stimuli facilitate movement and gait initiation and continuation.	−Auditory (earpiece with "beep") −Visual (Light flashes delivered with a light flashing diode) −Somatosensory (pulsed vibrations through a wrist band)
Formalized Patterned Exercises	Patterned and practiced movements aimed at improving balance and posture	−Tai chi −Qigong −Dance therapy

focused attention in patients with PD is not yet clear and needs further study. Cueing may not have a role for most patients with PD; however, there may be a subset (individuals who suffer from severe gait freezing and gait initiation) who benefit from this modality of therapy.[5]

Formalized patterned exercises (tai chi, qigong) as a therapy for PD have been studied in the past five years. These exercises are primarily focused on balance training, focusing attention, and improvement of flexibility. The results of several studies have been mixed as to the sustainability of the therapy and the clinical significance.[6,7] A 2012 study by Li et al. in a group of patients with predominantly mild to moderate PD comparing tai chi to resistance training and stretching showed that tai chi was an effective stand-alone therapy. Moreover, this was the first modality to demonstrate a reduction in falls in a population with PD of mild to moderate severity.[8] While more studies are needed of this modality, these results are encouraging.

The combined results of exercise and physical therapy indicate that patients with PD can benefit in multiple ways from participation in these forms of therapy. We encourage our patients to engage in these activities after diagnosis. There are recognized hurdles to these interventions that are difficult to assess in randomized controlled trials. Most trials occur in supervised centers, requiring patients to have the means or ability to regularly travel. There is a significant investment of time (several times a week in most studies) and money. Most of these therapies require relatively normal cognitive function. Finally, the goals of the intervention should be long-term—staving off long-term disability—however, the studies are frequently done over a short period of time (a few weeks to months). Home-based regimens may actually have higher adherence rates compared to center-based programs. In fact, adherence to the regimen may be the most important factor for any exercise-based therapy. Strategies to improve adherence to the regimen may be the most significant challenge to the clinician in using these therapies. Finally, patient safety must be taken into account at all times when engaging in any of these therapies.[9] Table 12.2 summarizes the benefits and challenges reviewed for physical therapy and PD.

Table 12.2 Benefits and Challenges in Using Physical Therapy Regimens in PD	
Benefits	**Challenges**
Improve motor UPDRS scores	Transportation to center-based programs
Improve gait metrics (speed, stride length, stride width)	Cost
	Adherence to regimen
Balance improvement	Safety during regimen
Efficacious as a symptomatic adjunct to levodopa	Difficulty for use in cognitively impaired patients
Possibly reduce risk of falls	Labor-intensive
Improved quality of life/outlook	Requires a motivated patient
Possibly improve mortality	Physical limitations (musculoskeletal pain a common cause for study dropout)
Possibly improve symptomatic gait freezing	

Occupational Therapy

The distinct benefits from occupational therapy separate from a combined re-habilitation program with occupational, physical, and speech therapy have not been adequately studied. Occupational therapy focuses on specific functional activities aimed at improving quality of life and improvement of skilled activities. Training of motor skills can be diverse, including balance, mobility, and object manipulation. Occupational therapists also focus on organization and process skills such as task sequence and adaptive skills. No clear type of occupational therapy has been determined effective; however, given the diverse nature of occupational therapy, it is difficult to study. Patients can derive a benefit and improvement in motor function and quality of life while they are participating in therapy. Moreover, occupational therapy has been shown to be safe and well tolerated by patients with PD. The most likely context for occupational therapy in the care of patients with PD is as part of a combination-therapy approach individualized to the patient and their specific needs.[1,10]

Speech Therapy

Speech dysfunction, manifested by hypophonia (soft voice) is a common impair-ment in patients with PD. For individuals who are employed, this can be a par-ticularly difficult problem as it commonly affects their ability to be heard on the telephone and speak in meetings or other gatherings. The Lee Silverman Voice Treatment (LSVT) is the most studied and effective therapy to date. It is an in-tensive therapy aimed at increasing phonatory effort and vocal cord adduction. Treatment is intensive, typically offered four times a week for four weeks.[11] Speech therapy using LSVT can improve hypophonia, and in two randomized trials, the improvement on speech volume was sustained for up to 24 months after therapy.[12,13] As an overall treatment for PD, LSVT has not been shown to improve UPDRS scores or overall motor function. However, as a targeted therapy for the specific impairment of hypophonia, it is an effective therapy for improving speech volume. Moreover, the sustained benefits after the intensive therapy session improve the effectiveness of the treatment.

Dysphagia is another common problem in PD for which speech therapy may be a useful symptomatic treatment. While most studies examining the effects of therapy on swallowing are small, with limited controls, there does appear to be a benefit in some groups of patients. The most studied modality is swallowing retraining. As in many forms of therapy, patients need to be cognitively intact to participate. This can present a challenge, as dysphagia is often a later complica-tion of PD when cognitive deficits frequently co-occur.

Summary

Delaying disability in Parkinson's disease can be approached in many different ways. Mild impairments such as hypophonia, reduced manual dexterity, or gait slowing may not be functionally disabling, but may cause enough impairment to

Table 12.3 An Integrated Approach to Rehabilitation Therapy in PD

Therapy	Goals	Utility in Symptomatic Improvement in PD
Physiotherapy: Exercise, Treadmill Training	Maintaining of gait function, preservation of balance, and delaying functional disability	Recommended after diagnosis of PD. In early PD, can be incorporated in a home-based setting.
Cueing and Focused Attention	Improvement in gait initiation and freezing	Can be considered in patients with symptomatic gait freezing.
Tai Chi/Qigong, Formalized Pattern Exercises	Maintenance of balance, may improve fall risk	Can be used in ambulatory patients with mild to moderate PD.
Occupational Therapy	Improvement of motor skills and adapting functional activities for improvement of quality of life	Most beneficial as part of a multidisciplinary approach in moderate and advanced PD.
Speech Therapy: LSVT Swallowing Retraining	Improved phonation and voice volume. Improvement of dysphagia	Symptom-specific for hypophonia. Can be recommended throughout PD course, often most useful for highly functional patients limited by this symptom.Symptom-specific for dysphagia; patients need to be cognitively intact.

make the individual reduce work and limit enjoyable activities, or may reduce the overall quality of life. Target therapies through rehabilitation specialists are available for treating these specific problems. Table 12.3 summarizes the role of the therapies described and how they are best utilized. More disabling problems such as balance impairment and falling serve as the leading edge of functional disability. Non-pharmacological therapies have the potential to delay this disability from gait dysfunction, which does influence mortality from PD. This is an active area of research, as researchers learn more about the relationship between disability, mortality, and disease progression in PD. We advise that all patients with PD be provided information about the options, goals, and effectiveness of these non-pharmacological treatments. While in the past these therapies may have been on the periphery of a patient's treatment regimen, they are now becoming a significant pillar in the multidisciplinary care of individuals with PD.[14]

References

1. Fox SH, Katenschlager R, Lim SY, et al. The Movement Disorder Society Evidence medical review update: treatments for the motor symptoms of Parkinson's disease. *Mov Disord.* 2011;26:S1–S41.

2. Shulman LM, Gurber-Baldini AL, Anderson KE, et al. The evolution of disability in Parkinson's disease. *Mov Disord.* 2008;23:790–796.

3. Morris ME, Iansek R, Kirkwood B. A randomized controlled trial of movement strategies compared with exercise for people with Parkinson's disease. *Mov Disord.* 2009;24:64–71.

4. Sage MD, Almeida QJ. Symptom and gait changes after sensory attention focused exercise vs. aerobic training in Parkinson's disease. *Mov Disord.* 2009;24:1132–1138.

5. Nieuwboer A, Kwakkel G, Rochester L, et al. Cueing training in the home improves gait-related mobility in Parkinson's disease: the RESCUE trial. *J Neurol Neurosurg Psychiatry.* 2007;78: 134–140.

6. Hackney ME, Earhart GM. Tai chi improves balance and mobility in people with Parkinson's disease. *Gait Posture.* 2008;28: 456–460.

7. Schmitz-Hubsch T, Pyfer D, Kielwein K, Fimmers R, Klockgether T, Wullner U. Qigong exercise for the symptoms of Parkinson's disease: a randomized, controlled pilot study. *Mov Disord.* 2006;21:543–548.

8. Li F, Harmer P, Fitzgerald K, et al. Tai chi and postural stability in patients with Parkinson's disease. *N Engl J Med.* 2012;366:511–519.

9. Allen NE, Sherrington C, Suriyarachchi GD, Paul SS, Song J, Canning CG. Exercise and motor training in people with Parkinson's disease: a systematic review of participant characteristics, intervention delivery, retention rates, adherence, and adverse events in clinical trials. *Parkinson's Dis,* vol. 2012, article ID 854328, 15 pages, 2012. doi:10.1155/2012/854328

10. Rao AK. Enabling functional independence in Parkinson's disease: update on occupational therapy intervention. *Mov Disord.* 2010;25:S146–S151.

11. Fox CM, Morrison CE, Ramig LO, Sapir S. Current perspectives on the Lee Silverman Voice Treatment (LSVT) for individuals with idiopathic Parkinson's disease. *Amer J Speech-Lang Pathol* 2002;11:111–123.

12. Ramig LO, Sapir S, Fox C, Countryman S. Changes in vocal loudness following intensive voice treatment (LSVT) in individuals with Parkinson's disease: a comparison with untreated patients and normal age-matched controls. *Mov Disord.* 2001;16:79–83.

13. Ramig LO, Sapir S, Countryman S, et al. Intensive voice treatment (LSVT) for patients with Parkinson's disease: a 2-year follow up. *J Neurol Neurosurg Psychiatry.* 2001;71:493–498.

14. Baijens LWJ, Speyer R. Effects of therapy for dysphagia in Parkinson's disease: systemic review. *Dsyphagia.* 2009;24:91–102.

Index

Tables, boxes and figures are indicated by an italic "t", "b", or "f" following the page number.

JUN 2 9 2015

Date Due
